Commit to Get Fit

Find the Secret to Your Own True and
Everlasting Weight Loss

Laura Dion-Jones

ISBN 978-0-9794914-3-6

Learn to —

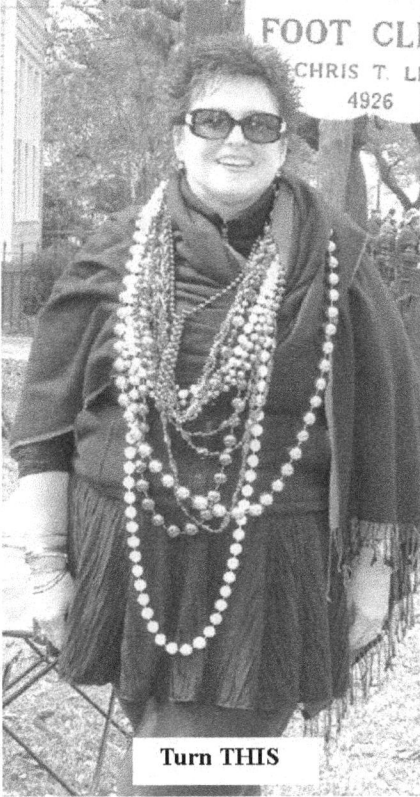

Turn THIS

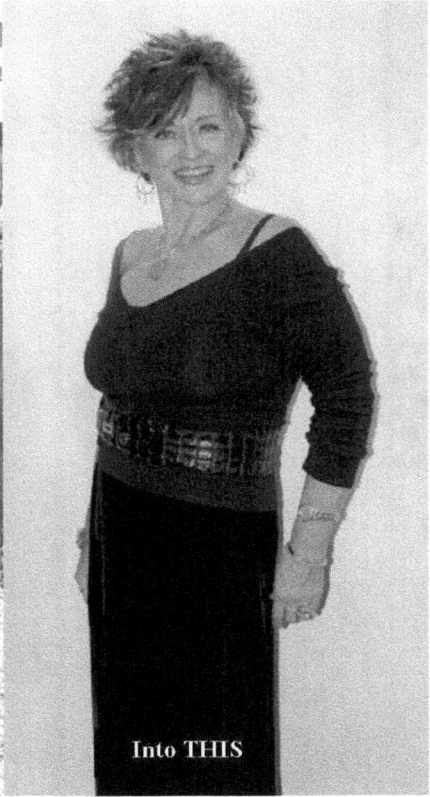

Into THIS

To Ellery Casey,

without whom none of this would be possible.

Thank you from my heart.

Table of Contents

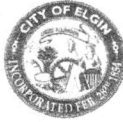

David J. Kaptain
MAYOR

150 DEXTER COURT
ELGIN, ILLINOIS 60120

847/931-5595
mayor@cityofelgin.org

November 20, 2013

As the mayor of Elgin, Illinois, I remember well when Laura Dion-Jones first brought her "Commit to Get Fit" program to town. I not only was a guest on her weekly radio show several times, but I also saw firsthand the positive things she was doing in the community.

Laura's level of pro-health advocacy set fitness as a lifelong goal. She talked openly and publicly about facing obesity herself in earlier years, coming across as a regular woman who needed a road to wellness as much as a way to get there. Her way became a success story that included healthier eating habits and an absolute dedication to daily walking, something I also strongly believe in. In addition, she introduced a popular fitness initiative, course and competition called "Elgin's Biggest Loser," during which she helped dozens and dozens of men and women lose hundreds and hundreds of pounds. She would tell them that we can change only what we are willing to face and acknowledge. She created weight loss plans designed for real people living real lives. And she did it with a smile on her face and the best interest of others at heart.

Laura Dion-Jones is an asset to anyone or any group looking for an accountability-based fitness program. She was a catalyst toward better health for many men and women in our area. As mayor, I'm grateful for that. And I'm grateful for the positive energy she brought to Elgin.

Sincerely,

David J. Kaptain
Mayor

Introduction

Hey, Fat Ass!

The shout from the back of the passing truck pierced my heart and the lovely fall day's crisp air as I waited to cross Rush Street with my two little dogs in tow.

Some guy evidently didn't like the way I looked and felt the need to insult me. He had it right, however, because I didn't like the way I looked, either. And I had no idea what to do about it.

Are you sick of being fat?

I certainly was. I couldn't stand it another freaking second. After living a lifetime in chronic obesity's shoes—enough was enough.

Scared out of my mind because I really had no idea what to do next, I had a much-needed "Come-to-Jesus" talk with myself. What finally clicked for me was that I needed to wake up from my food-induced coma before it was too late. At 317 pounds, my weight was rapidly escalating and I knew I really needed to change my life to save my life. I needed to find a way out of chronic obesity's hell once and for all.

Actually, there's a bit more to it than this, but, besides the major catastrophic health issues I faced at this weight, what clicked for me was that I was sick of being sick and sick of being tired.

I was sick of being fat.

I was sick of hauling myself around.

I was sick of being out of breath at every turn.

I was sick of looking like a blimp in clothing no matter how fabulous or flattering the design, no matter how chic, expensive, or unique the outfit (always my design from my Dion-Jones, Ltd. plus-size fashion label, of course: www.dionjonesltd.com!), no matter how wonderful I looked.

I was sick of being the fattest one in the room, the fattest one in the crowd, the fattest one in the entire place.

I was sick of being looked at either in admiration (I always made sure I looked like a movie star no matter how big I got—it was my only defense and the only thing I was able to control) or looked at in disgust because I was so big, but looked sharper than anyone else around. I'd occasionally hear, "How dare such a big, fat, slob look so fabulous?" I might have been big and I might have been fat, but I assure you I was no slob.

I was sick of always being told how utterly beautiful I was " … if only you'd lose a little weight."

I was sick of being called names that had absolutely nothing to do with me as a person, nothing to do with my talents and creativity, and nothing whatsoever to do with my expertise and performance in my various successful professions.

Exceptional Contemporary High Fashion to Flatter the Fuller Figure.

Sizes 12 to Super Size 60
in Petite - Average or Tall

I was sick of whispering to the flight attendant, "Can I please use a seatbelt extender?" as I got on the plane and then covertly slipping it back into her hand as I disembarked.

I was sick of the overly

theatric, humiliatingly disparaging looks and comments I received from WASP-y nineteen-year-old boys, on two separate occasions, at major collection showings at Chicago's Art Institute. Who would expect such ridiculous size prejudice existed in that cultured, rarified air?

On a visit to Frank Lloyd Wright's beloved Taliesin in Wisconsin, I was beyond mortified when I heard one of the gift shop clerks hiss into her phone to one of her colleagues in another department, "You've got to come up here and see something that will be very cleansing for you." I knew she was talking about me, and I didn't know whether to shit, shoot, or go blind in embarrassment.

And did I mention that it was getting increasingly difficult for me to move, to climb stairs, and to get in and out of a car, let alone buckle the seat belt around one of my gorgeous, but a little bit bulkier coats? "Hmm. This darn coat has gotten just a bit too cumbersome," I'd complain, when in reality, I was the one who had gotten a bit too cumbersome for my own good.

The Perfect Storm

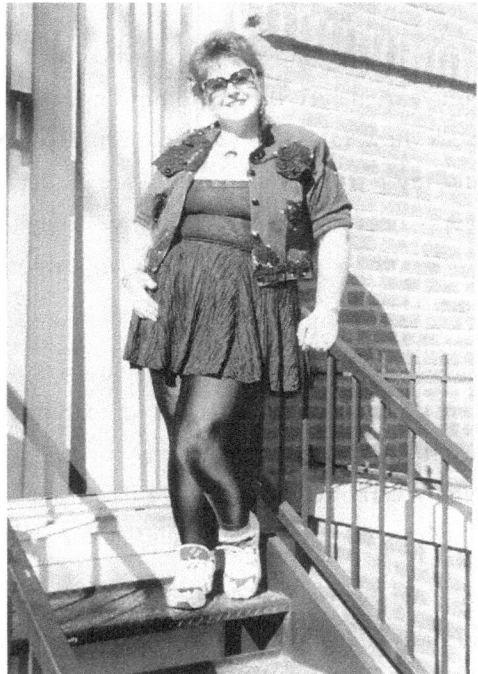

Suddenly, all of these circumstances and a few more came crashing together, culminating in my own personal "Perfect Storm." When I realized the storm was inside of me, something clicked. I had had enough. *I decided to stop making excuses for my eating and to take responsibility for every morsel I put into my mouth from that moment on.*

You're fat because you eat too much and/or drink too much of the wrong things. You're fat because you do not move nearly enough. Period. No more excuses. No more denial. No more cons. No more nothin'.

Sure, some of us have physical and structural issues to deal with. Some have thyroid, insulin, hormonal, or glandular problems that help keep us fat, too. Whatever the case, it's your individual responsibility to get those things checked out with a good endocrinologist and/or appropriate doctor. If you really want to lose weight, you'll find a safe, healthy way. Obesity and poor health are realities, but they no longer have to be an issue. Obesity and poor health also know no prejudice and have no bounds. Unfortunately, society has a prejudice against overweight people no matter how rich, famous, or powerful they are. Plus, being obese is just plain unhealthy. And unnecessary. And totally, unequivocally preventable.

A Last-Ditch Effort to Get Yourself Back from Obesity's Brink

If you're the kind of person who gains weight just by looking at food, if you've tried everything and nothing has worked *in the long term*, then a five-week, how-to, quick-start "Commit to Get Fit" health and fitness program and my terrific how-to advice are all detailed for you in this book. It's five weeks because it takes thirty-five straight days to make or break a habit. *Make this the year you begin to lose weight once and for all, and I'll show you how.*

Recent expert statistics claim that diets aren't working. Baloney, I say, and here's why: the "experts" need to redefine *healthy eating*, because what's healthy for some isn't healthy for everyone—especially for those who are highly carbohydrate sensitive like I am. If you constantly struggle to lose weight, what most experts suggest may not be healthy for you, either.

In listening to the medical and media professionals spout their mostly outdated diet dogmas, the majority of them tout the same old, same old, which never worked for me and obviously isn't working for you or the other overweight people across our nation, either.

The latest medical buzz is that the Mediterranean Diet is the best diet above all others. I will tell you this: it didn't work well enough for me—regardless of the proposed health benefits—to continue struggling on it to lose weight. Which I didn't.

Why? Because I'm extremely hyperinsulinemic, which means I overproduce insulin in a huge way. Insulin is a hormone secreted by the pancreas that ultimately controls fat storage. The legumes and certain higher-glycemic fruit that nutritional experts recommend on some diets actually retard my weight loss every single step of the way. If you're highly carb sensitive like me, your pancreas doesn't care if it's an Idaho potato or a sweet potato—unlike the pancreatic function of naturally thinner, "normal" folks. The only thing your pancreas knows is that you're fueling it with starch and sugar, and it will push out more than enough insulin to compensate. But in those of us who are hyperinsulinemic, it's the overproduction of insulin that makes us fat and keeps us that way. Not dietary fat.

I have to eat low-glycemic foods regardless of the complexity of the carb— my pancreas cannot seem to distinguish between simple and complex carbohydrates. And I firmly believe it's this way for nearly all obese people across the board, making it the biggest reason there is an obesity epidemic in our country. Of course, many, many other factors enter into it, but I strongly believe this is the root reason of obesity today.

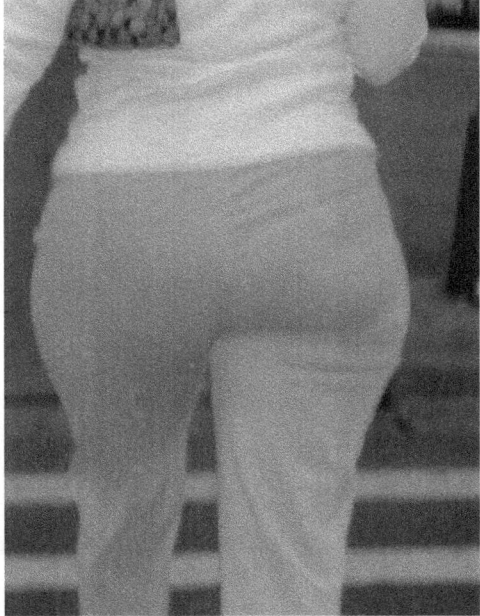

Are You Carb Sensitive?

Think about it. You can easily test your sensitivity to carbohydrates, just like I did. Try it. But when you do, come from a place of 100% integrity in your efforts. No cheating. However, the only way to truly evaluate the consequences and risks of eating the wrong foods is to also factor your daily exercise regime (or lack thereof) into your research results. Only then will you know exactly what works for your personal weight loss and what doesn't.

Keep a food and fitness journal for a month. Proposed journal research entries can include:

- Here's what happened when I ate _____ (fill in the blank with a certain type of food) for so many days in a row:

- Here's what happened when I *didn't* eat _____ (fill in the blank with the same type of food) for so many days in a row:

- Here's what happened when I did my cardio for thirty-five straight days:_____ (fill in the blank about your experience)

Hopefully, your cardio entry would read something along the lines of: "I got addicted to it. First I hated it. And then I began to crave it; if I didn't squeeze in (at least) a thirty-minute walk by the time my lunch hour was over, I didn't feel right. WTF happened to me? I was never like this before! I loved sitting around and gossiping with the gang after lunch, but gossiping never made me look or feel this good."

After picking a diet* you can live with for the rest of your life, think of your new eating plan as the lifestyle you have to live with forever, *not* as just another diet. Almost instantly, you'll become much healthier when you practice making better food choices, but you have to also add a few simple changes—with the emphasis on *simple*. You'll also need to learn how to exercise portion control. Then add an hour of serious daily cardio into the mix and you're on your way.*

You'll begin to realize that you are totally in control of your life and your future. Only you. Knowing you are on your way to attaining your goals because you are able to, because you *want to,* rather than because you *have to,* makes a huge difference in the way you continue to move forward. When you are in control of every morsel that you put into your mouth and how you move, the obstacles that stand in your way become challenges you can overcome, and your journey starts to be an adventure instead of a prison sentence. I know the prison sentence all too well, which is detailed in the first part of this book. I hope my story and understanding the science behind lasting weight loss will inspire you.

Your new you is waiting.

Your future is in your hands.

Stop stumbling into the future. Create your own.

And don't worry, it's much easier than you think, but do choose your diet and daily cardio plans wisely. You're going to be in this healthier rut for the rest of your life, so you might as well learn to enjoy it. Your main goal is doing all of these things everyday in order to make them lifelong habits, so that you actually crave them when you don't practice daily. Keeping yourself healthy for the rest of your life is your end-game strategy. To change your lifestyle, you have to be in it for the long haul—to win it.

Once you define your diet and begin your daily cardio, you'll begin to lose weight. You'll also feel satisfied and energized, no longer hungry, sloppy, and sluggish. And if you do find yourself feeling like this, then you'll know you're not on the right diet for you. Every pound you lose should empower you.

Tell the truth about where you're at right now with your weight and what you eat. And then believe you can actually be successful this time in your dieting and daily exercise efforts, no matter how many times you've tried in the past. It's a brand-new day with a brand-new you waiting on the horizon.

Need a jumpstart?

Keep reading, because if you quit now, you'll never win.

*As with any new diet and fitness plan, be sure to check with your physician before you begin.

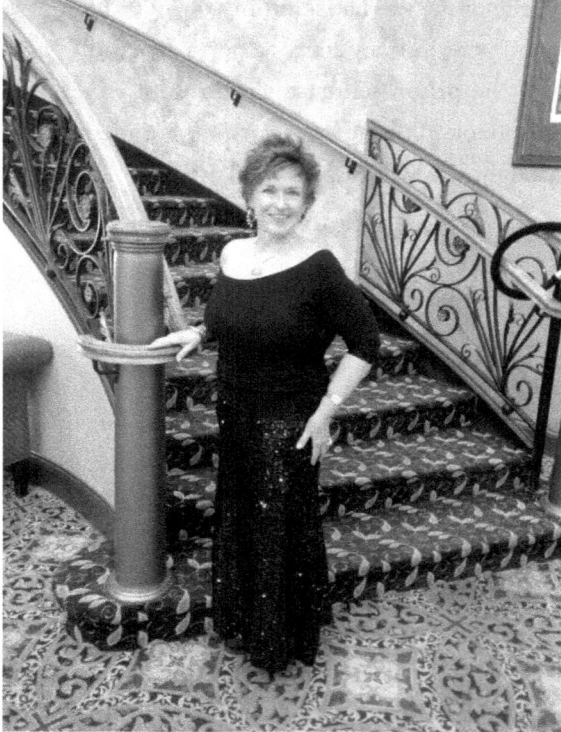

Part One

My Weight-Loss Story

Chapter 1

The Magic Number for Me: 317

"Life demands from you the strength that you possess. Only one feat is possible—not to have run away."

—Dag Hammarskjold, Swedish statesman and Secretary-General of the United Nations

When I woke up from my food-induced coma over ten years ago, I found myself at an all-time high of 317 pounds—and climbing. I was mortified beyond belief. I knew that if I didn't stop the scale's ascent and reverse my weight's direction immediately, I'd be dead before I knew it. This was the third time in my life my weight had skyrocketed to the 300-pound stratosphere. Enough was enough.

People wonder, and sometimes I do, too, how I let my weight get that far out of hand. The truth is, at the time I had no idea how to actually stop it. I didn't understand the importance of daily cardio and I certainly didn't realize the impact foods heavy in white starch and sugar carbs had on my mind, body, and system.

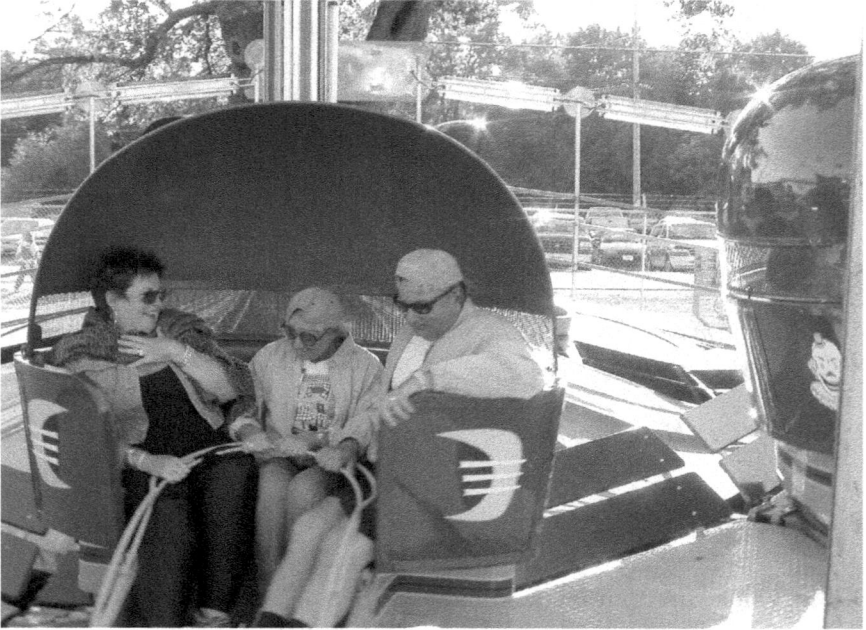

How I Got to 317 Pounds

Once upon a time, I was considered a black-run skier. I loved every second of whizzing down a mountain or even a Midwest mole hill and absolutely lived to ski. Actually, when it was time to ski, I would rather ski than eat—stopping to grab some lunchtime liquid refreshment and getting back out on the slopes as fast as possible was of utmost importance to me. Back then, my record for skiing Aspen was about seven times in one winter.

I was one of the top hair and makeup artists in the Midwest, working my butt off twelve to eighteen hours a day, three to four days a week, and was able to arrange my work schedule to suit my skiing passion. In February of 2002, we were skiing Steamboat Springs, Colorado, another absolutely heavenly skiers' paradise. And as was my custom at the end of the day, I would egg everyone on to take all the lifts and gondolas to the very top of the mountain so that we could ski down with the ski patrol, getting our last run in. Ahhh, I can smell the piñon- and pine-scented air as we speak.

It was one of those incredibly sublime ski days, where the sun was shining brightly, not a cloud in the deep azure-blue sky, and the snow was semi-soft like a freshly shaved snow cone. We wore our jackets tied around our waists, no hats, gloves, goggles, nothing extra to get in the way of enjoying that last run. This was pre-spring skiing at its very best in years.

And, as you may have heard, it's always the very last run of the day ...

As usual, I led the way from the very top as we all pointed our skis down a freshly groomed black run. About a third of the way down, I was cruising into a soft-arc turn, when I spotted a beginning skier panicked out of his shorts, snowplowing his way right straight toward me with his poles waving around wildly like runaway plane propellers. It was obvious that this young man was in way over his ski tips.

As soon as it dawned on me that he was out of control, heading straight toward me, I yelled at him, "Move your poles!" and in that split second, pantomimed drawing my own poles into my sides so he'd get the hint about what to do. No such luck. As I carved into my turn, one of his poles had gotten stuck smack in the middle of my right binding, sending me into a fall. As I slowly went down I felt a burn so intense in my right knee that all I could think of was, *WTF is going on here?* It literally felt like a blowtorch was shooting flames that were focused squarely on my right knee.

In total disbelief, I watched helplessly as my knee wrenched right out of the socket. Instead of my leg being at, say, twelve o'clock high from the knee down to the tip of my ski, it was now aiming straight up hill as if pointing to three o'clock, away from the rest of my body—which, BTW, was the name of my final, fatal run: Three O'Clock.

The whole thing happened so fast that my husband, who was right behind me, was unable to stop to help and shot right past. He screeched to a halt a short distance downhill from where I was lodged and yelled, "Should I go get the ski patrol?"

"Yes!" I screamed as I slid sideways and ever so slowly down the slope. The pain was so off the charts that all I wanted was for it to stop. I still could not comprehend what was happening to me. I had absolutely no idea a knee could actually bend to the side at a 90-degree angle like that.

I am told the young man who caused this catastrophic collision composed himself and continued to snowplow slowly down the rest of the hill, poles still whirling in every direction like twin helo-rotors sucking for air, leaving me there to fend for myself.

By the time the ski patrol arrived with the body-sized rescue basket that would be my transport to the emergency room at the base of the mountain, quite a crowd had gathered. The severity of my injury had not penetrated my brain past the intense pain. The entire back of my body felt every single ripple, bump, blip, stone, and piece of balled up ice and snow that my basket slid over as we made our way down the mountain. At one point I remember hearing the lead rescue sled skier say they had to load my basket—with me in it—onto a ski lift because the runs were far too dangerous for any of them to ski me all the way down to the bottom. *This I have to see,* I thought.

I didn't realize that due to the severity of my injury, and because they were almost certain everything in my knee was shredded to smithereens, the ski patrol's main concern was whether or not my femoral artery was also torn. If that was the case, I had a limited amount of time before my leg would be without blood flow and there was a great possibility I could lose it.

We've all seen those pro ball boys roll around the field or court when they tear one of their ligaments. Well, all mine were absolutely ripped to bits, so multiply an ACL tear by four and you'll get the picture.

Once in the emergency room at base camp, the head nurse came toward me wielding a pair of scissors and a wicked gleam in her eye, making a beeline straight for my ski pants. I knew exactly what she was going to do and I told her there was absolutely no way in hell she was gonna cut my custom-made ski pants off me. As one of the country's first and top plus-size designers and models from the early 1980s to the late 1990s, I designed those pants and even imported the special wool and Lycra fabric straight from the manufacturer that made the jodhpurs for the Royal Canadian Mounted Police (I swear). So there was no way in the world that I was gonna let that babe cut those pants off me (as if I'd ever ski again, but I didn't know it at the time).

With that, the nurse scurried off in a huff to get the doctor. One thing led to another and, before I knew what hit me, he snuck up and gave me about three shots of morphine to shut me up. When I awoke a bit later, my ski pants were off—and still intact, I might add—and my leg was now straight and encased in a serious immobilizing brace with a zillion straps holding it in place from my heel to the top of my thigh.

"Nice work, Doc," I remember half joking as I came to and watched him busily doing other necessary things for and around me. Then the doctor asked me some personal questions, but the one that really caught my attention was, "So, how long did it take you to finish your triathlon?" His question puzzled me because I didn't remember telling him anything about my triathlon. (Read "Going the Distance" in chapter 20.)

Turns out that morphine is like truth serum, and after he shot me, I evidently blabbed my brains out about my triathlon experience while he and his team straightened out my leg, then slid my ski pants off so they could do what they needed to do to get me ready to be sent off in a private Learjet to St. Anthony's Hospital in Denver, the best and closest place for me to get an angiogram of my right leg. They had to make sure the femoral artery was still intact. If it wasn't, I stood a good chance of losing my leg. And here I was getting all pissy with them about my custom ski pants.

Thankfully, the angiogram revealed that the one and only thing left intact in my leg was my femoral artery. *Thank God!* I wasn't up for the challenge of living the rest of my life without my right leg. Before the doctors at St. Anthony's would release me, I had to learn how to maneuver up and down an entire flight of stairs on crutches with military precision—because I was going to be in that condition, on those crutches, indefinitely.

That turned out to be the easy part. Once back in Chicago, the real test began: I had to find an orthopedic surgeon to put me back together and help me heal. I saw eight doctors before I settled on the right one. Yes, eight. Numbers one through six each gave me a different song and dance and treatment option. It was quite confusing to hear all those different opinions; I didn't know which way to turn.

Finally, out of frustration, I called Freddy Cato, the head trainer of the Chicago Bears football team at the time. I introduced myself and told him what had happened to me and asked, "If I were your star quarterback, and this happened, what would you do to help me?" Thankfully, he took pity on me and told me to be in River Forest the following morning at 9:00 a.m. to see the head doctor for the Bears.

Dr. Berna told me, "Your knee is so inflamed right now, it's like an abscessed tooth. We can do nothing for you until the swelling and inflammation go down. Mild daily physical therapy would be best for you at this time." I left his office feeling a bit relieved because things finally made sense.

On the way home from Dr. Berna's office, I was crying, whining, sick of telling my ski accident story over and over and over to each and every doctor, lawyer, resident, and receptionist. My husband encouraged me to not give up and keep my appointment with Dr. Hill. He came very highly recommended, and the next day I did just that.

Some of the other doctors I'd seen were quite arrogant, and I didn't like the way they treated me or what they told me. I got the impression that a few of them were just trying to give me the bum's rush and slap me into surgery too quickly. Nothing the first six doctors told us made any sense. That's why I kept going from one to the next to the next.

Dr. Berna was doctor number seven; Dr. Jimmy Hill from Northwestern University Hospital was number eight. He entered the exam room with his right hand outstretched and one of the biggest, most genuine smiles I'd ever seen. His lab coat read Dr. James Hill, M.D., Orthopedics. Were it not for that, you'd never know he was such an incredible doctor and a master at his craft. "Hi, I'm Jimmy Hill, let's see what we have here?" he kindly stated.

Dr. Hill has performed countless knee scopes on my right knee since that day we first met. Then as my weight packed on by the handfuls, my left knee eventually gave out, so the scopes began on that knee, too.

As is the case when you really don't know better, I was mystified and panicked at my declining state of health. The heavier I got, the harder it was for me to move. And all the while, I was in and out of physical therapy, rehabbing from the latest knee surgery or some other physical issue or ailment—mostly due to the fact I was getting increasingly fatter by the New York nanosecond. Why mince words?

I watched helplessly as the numbers on that damn scale rose higher, and higher, and higher the "healthier" I ate. Throughout the rest of this book , I happily and humbly share with you the story of my journey back to health and wellness and how I finally found the Secret To My Own True And Everlasting Weight Loss.

I can't caution you enough about how severely your excess weight impacts your physical, mental, personal, and professional lives—more than you'll ever know—until you get it off and keep it off forever. Once you realize and taste what it's like to be a thinner, lighter, healthier, more beautiful, and fit person, there ain't no goin' back—at least there wasn't for me.

I always tell everyone I have no choice but to continue my health and fitness quest every single day I have left on this planet, as long as I'm able to move down my lane on the healthy highway of life. And you know what everyone tells me? I did have a choice and I still have a choice; I choose health and better fitness over being obese and hobbled by food ever again. Being obese is SO not worth it, kids.

I hope my personal story helps inspire you to let me help you *Find the Secret to Your Own True and Everlasting Weight Loss* once and for all, just like I did. I saw firsthand what it was like to stare into the belly of the obesity beast and also what it was like to be mildly handicapped. I knew I had to do something about it—and soon.

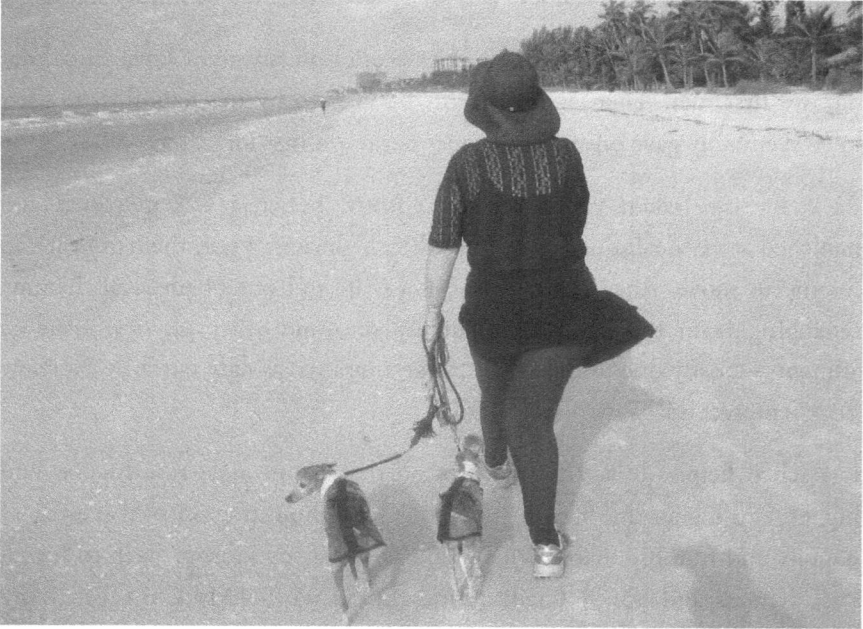

Each one of my medical professionals listed in the back of this book loves me. They respect me for my extreme efforts, daily diligence, and hypermotivation in spite of all the physical challenges I face on a daily basis. And they know that when I say I did something, they can believe me. If I say I didn't, you can take that to the bank, too.

One more thing: You can ask anyone who belongs to or works at Chicago's East Bank Club and at Athletico Physical Therapy's outpost in the club about my daily dedication and discipline. They've all seen me hobble over to the club one week after every knee surgery, scope, replacement, and such. They've all seen me come on crutches, using a cane, limping, working out, and doing whatever it takes to move my body down the street each and every day. I'm told I'm an incredible role model and motivator, an inspiration to all - just because I'm there striving every single day. It's not just that I walk the walk and walk the talk, I truly feel there is absolutely no other way to live. For me. For you. For anyone and everyone with weight issues.

One of the biggest morals to this story: always, always, always get another medical opinion when you're in doubt or when what doctors tell you doesn't make sense to you. Just like finding the right mate, a great restaurant, or even a terrific hairdresser, it's the same for finding someone who's going to help you save your life.

And never, never, never, ever give up. Wherever there's a will, you have to find a way to lose your unhealthy, unwanted weight once and for all. I can help you. Keep reading.

And to quote the great Mikki Williams, CSP, CPAE, internationally famous speaking professional, coach, and mentor: "It all comes down to choice management, *not* time management. Own it. You have the time, make the choice."

And as our very favorite Auntie Mame says: "Life is a banquet and most poor suckers are starving to death." Being overweight isn't starving to death for food, but it sure is starving to death because you're missing out on so much of life.

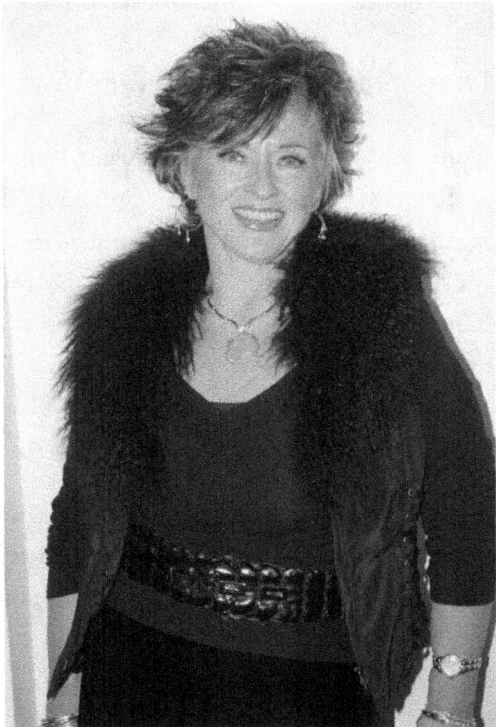

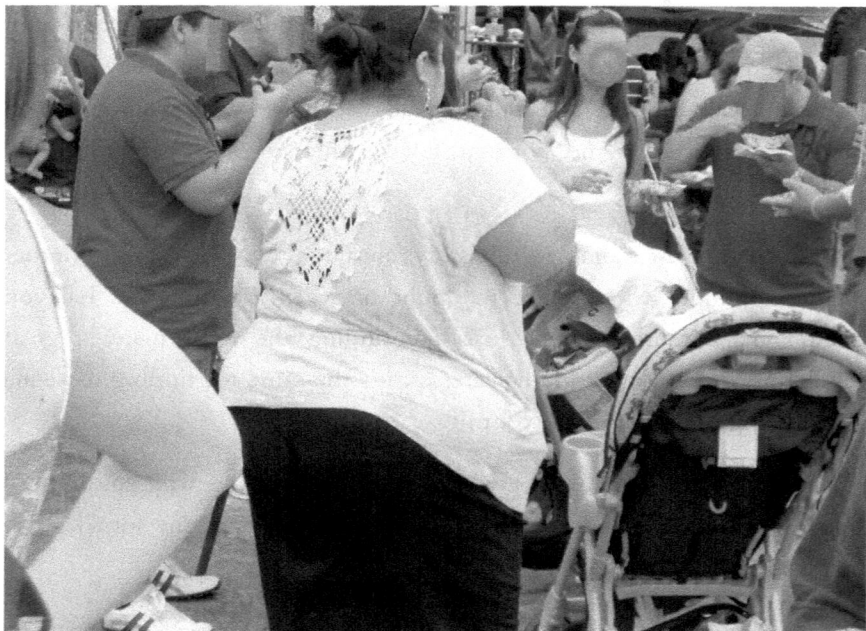

Desperate Strategies Never Work

Desperate, I tried all the old weight-loss strategies that had worked for me in the past. I bought every diet book that I could find; visited highly regarded, registered nutritionists; experimented with hypnotherapy. I even consulted with the chairperson of the psychology department at a major university here in Chicago and nothing worked. The weight kept piling on by the handfuls. Convinced I had grown too weak for self-discipline, I resigned myself to having absolutely no way to lose weight other than by getting a gastric bypass or a gastric Lap-Band® procedure.

At the time I was considering these two drastic intestinal alterations, there were four nationally renowned doctors in the field of gastric bypass surgery. The physician's name that seemed to be on everyone's lips for the Midwest was right here in Chicago at one of our university hospitals. I always believe in going to the top, the best for whatever it is that I need, especially when it's medical, so I picked up the phone.

Deciding to go ahead with the bypass surgery was the easy part. After that, I had a hell of a time getting an appointment for the initial interview and intense multiple physical and psychological screenings necessary to be considered for the procedure.

Then the economy changed. Now, a lot of doctors will perform gastric bypasses and lap-bands on just about anyone who has insurance or money to cover the price of the procedure. I know a doctor who performed a gastric bypass on a woman who only needed to lose forty measly pounds. Sad and unconscionable, and not at all the easy way to weight-loss salvation most people hope for.

At the time I was contemplating a gastric bypass, all the available consultation slots were jammed with other desperate, anxious applicants. It seemed as if everyone in town that was the least bit overweight was already in line. I begged. I cajoled. I even tried to bribe the appointment scheduler with a two-week stay at our Florida vacation home if she'd squeeze me in earlier than the three-month-long wait list (no dice, though I always figure it doesn't hurt to try). Eventually, however, I was able to appeal to the softer side of the program's director, and within a day or two, I received a call that there had been a cancellation for one of the preliminary screening appointments. Could I be there in two weeks? I couldn't spit the word "Yes" out of my mouth fast enough.

One criterion for acceptance into the gastric bypass program at this particular university hospital was that the doctor had to be convinced beyond a shadow of a doubt, in the personal interview portion of the screening, that I had not been able to lose weight in any other way over the past three years. *Three years,* I thought. *Ha! Try ten years. Try a lifetime.* The doctor also didn't like the fact that I was "only 317 pounds" (at 5'7"). He was accustomed to working with people much more obese—the 450-pounders and up. I told him that I felt being fat was all relative and that it was pretty evident that I couldn't lose weight on my own. In the end, I convinced him I needed outside help—specifically, his surgical salvation's intervention.

Once I had completed the other required screenings and psychological evaluations necessary to become a bypass surgery candidate, I felt almost relieved. Something positive was finally going to happen with my now out-of-control weight. I could actually see a sliver of light at the end of that long, dark tunnel. And it wasn't the headlight of a speeding train, either. It was a glimmer of H-O-P-E.

Along with my acceptance into the gastric bypass program came a surgery date scheduled for the beginning of that January—six whole months away. If they had told me they could squeeze me in for my bypass procedure the very next day, I would have gladly hopped on the operating table at 6:00 a.m. and let them have at me. But six months? Yikes! Lord only knew how much more my weight would escalate through the holidays if left to my own devices. That was way too much time to think, way too much time to overeat. Again, I begged and pleaded to get in sooner, but was told I'd have to wait in line for a surgery cancellation, if there even was such a thing, and, as luck would have it, I was number two on *that* list. End of discussion.

As further preparation for the procedure and to answer some of our questions, the gastric bypass team invited me and a couple other pre-op candidates to attend a few sessions of the post-op support group that met once a month. I leapt at the chance. Tons of questions that needed clarification were whizzing around in my head, and I also wanted to see what had made everyone else who'd had this procedure so successful at losing their weight. *It couldn't all be from the surgery,* I thought. One support group meeting was all it took to convince me that a gastric bypass was not the magic bullet that would ensure my true and everlasting weight loss success.

There were several people at the support group meeting I attended who had experienced tremendous success with their surgeries. Some of the attendees were post-op one month, some up to two years and counting. Most disturbingly, there were some who had suddenly and mysteriously stopped losing weight twelve and thirteen months past their surgeries. Their appetites came back—especially cravings for the sweets and breads and other white, starchy, sugary carbs that had been their downfall and had gotten them into trouble with their weight in the first place—and, boy, were they ever panicked. Listening to their stories gave me the chills. I was terrified for them, too.

One young woman, who was thirteen months post-op, was crying—literally sobbing her eyes out—and between her tears she told us that she had recently stopped losing weight. Her weight had been at a standstill for over a month; she was now able to eat larger quantities of food than she had been able to eat since her surgery; and she kept obsessively checking her weight, hopping on and off the scale five, eight, even ten times a day. She was absolutely beside herself and didn't know what to do. Nothing she tried seemed to work for her anymore.

Another guy chimed in that he was having the same problems. He was even drinking two of his meals a day in protein shake form and couldn't understand his lack of weight loss, either. Again, his appetite for all the white starch and sugar, the foods that had gotten him into trouble to begin with, had returned. His stomach could now hold more food than it had right after his bypass and he reluctantly obliged. His eating had returned to where it had been before his surgery. He was freaked out of his mind.

During the final minutes of the discussion, the doctor who had performed all the gastric bypass procedures at that hospital slipped into the meeting room. All eyes suddenly turned to him and silence fell over the group. Apparently he had been listening from the next room before he entered, because he started in without missing a beat.

"The secret to true and everlasting weight loss," he scolded, "if you haven't figured it out by now, is to starve yourself and exercise. A lot. You have to simply eat less, like you should've been doing over the past year, and you have to move more than you've been moving."

So, it all does boil down to one's will power, I thought. It was like an alarm going off in my head. Why go through all of the discomfort, pain, misery, and inconvenience of the surgery aftermath for one year, not to mention the expense, only to have to do the very same things you should have and could have been doing to lose weight in the first place, all on your own.

I knew it was time for me to go; this wasn't for me. As I left the room, so did the girl that had been crying about her waning weight loss. We shared the elevator on our way out and she asked me what I thought of the meeting. So, I told her honestly: "It scared me. You're no better off today than you were the day before your surgery. A year's passed and you still haven't taken the bull by the horns and developed all those skills you need to change your life and make new eating and exercise habits a part of your forever lifestyle. This is not something I want to do right now. There has to be another, better way."

The girl became enraged at my audacity, but the truth was, even though she had lost something like 145 pounds over the last year (dropping her to my exact weight at the time), she could lose no more. She simply didn't know how. For the first time, it became crystal clear. Saying those words out loud to her told me what I had to do for myself, and I nixed the bypass surgery idea altogether.

I was pretty scared leaving the hospital that day—the doctor dashing my hopes for my own surgical salvation, then my conversation in the elevator with the angry, crying young woman. I couldn't help but wonder where the program's nutritionists and counselors had been for her and some of the others struggling over the past year. I had previously gone the nutritionist route a few times myself, to no avail. It seemed white, starchy, sugary carbs were my archenemies; they sent my pancreas into overdrive, slowing me down and making me sleepy.

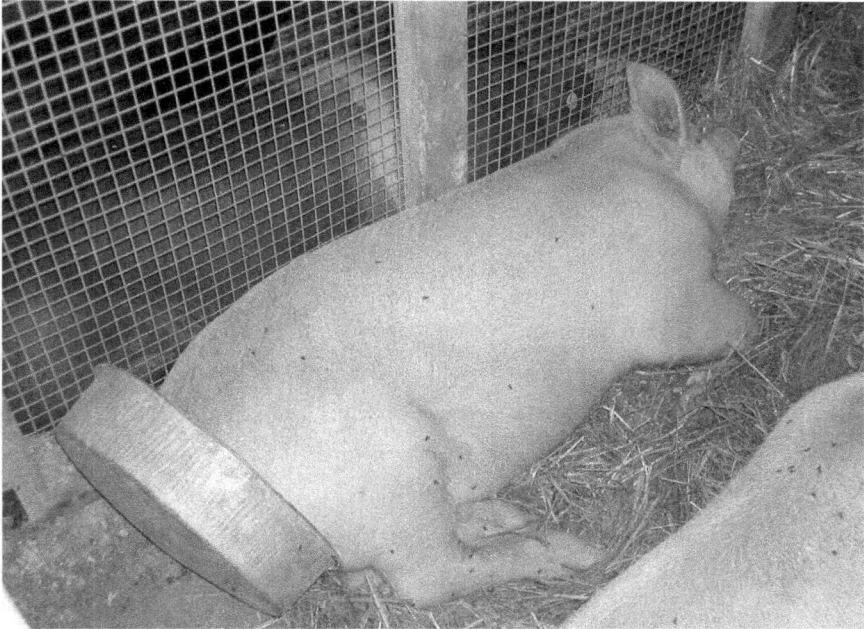

Carb Coma:
This is what happens when you eat too many white starch and sugar carbs.

Everything Else I Tried

Both of the top two nutritionists I had worked with here in Chicago believed in a low-fat diet along with that dang, carb-laden food group pyramid. Even with Weight Watchers, I'd never had much success because of the amount of carbs I was allowed in a day. White, starchy, sugary carbs, I found out shortly thereafter, are like poison for me and for many others like me.

Meanwhile, a good friend of mine had been bugging me for months to have my thyroid checked. "Oh, yeah, Carol," I'd say, "every fat person I know of on the face of the Earth is just *waiting* for their doctor to tell them that they have a thyroid problem, or that it's glandular, or that it's not their fault that they're so damn fat."

Carol refused to let up. She suspected something was wrong with me because she knew my eating habits first-hand. We'd shared many dinners, trips, and outings with our dogs, and she'd never really seen me overeat or snack my butt off enough to be as fat as I was. Plus, I was always cold no matter what the weather is. Same with my husband; he certainly was privy to my daily eating habits, knew I wasn't a closet eater, and he couldn't figure out my weighty situation, either.

Also, I wasn't a binger like some overweight people I know. I've never been the type to devour a half-gallon of ice cream or an entire cake or pie at one sitting. I absolutely can't relate to that—it would take me several days or up to a week to knock off any one of those things. If one consumes an entire small cheesecake over the course of five days, is that considered binging? I wasn't sure. But make no mistake: while I wasn't a binger, I packed away enough pasta, oatmeal, baked potatoes, rice and other *low-fat, "healthy"* foods and white starches and sugars to keep me fat for most of my life.

By the time I got home from the gastric bypass support group meeting, Carol had sent me another e-mail with a link to a site for "Top Endocrinologists in Your Area." This was only the fifth time she had needled me to find a new doctor, because my current doctor thought I just needed "a good diet and some exercise" and offered no help or advice beyond the same old, same old—which never, ever worked for me in the first place.

The stories I could tell you about the doctors I consulted would curl your eyelashes. A noted Ph.D., who specializes in nutrition and appears weekly on local TV, told me (with a straight face, mind you) "There's no such thing as willpower," when I sat in her office week after week, begging her to help me find mine.

Another doctor said that the reason I couldn't lose weight with his method was that I was probably repressing some childhood sexual abuse thing. In his experience, he claimed, "This was *always* the case." Not true, thank you. I did regression therapy and there's no evidence there. Oh, and one of my very favorites ever—the shrink (excuse me, chair of psychology at another local university hospital) who told me that I obviously *enjoyed* being so fat and that he could tell by the way I dressed and made myself up that I was way too proud of myself. "Otherwise, why would you go to such lengths to make yourself look so attractive and still be so fat? Even your jewelry and expensive perfume tell me you're way too proud of yourself," he hissed.

"Shoot, man, what do you consider 'too proud'?" I snarled back in his face. "How about making the best of the hand you've been dealt while you struggle to figure it all out?" Tearfully grabbing my bag, I raced out of his office as fast as my two proud, fat little feet could carry me. These are just a few of my "doctor experiences," in addition to all of the professional nutritionists, diet coaches, and sadistic trainers I consulted. I spent thousands of dollars on these people. And now Carol was suggesting I find yet another one. *Gee, thanks, Carol. You're kidding, right?*

Chapter 2

A New Beginning

"Don't just stumble into the future. You create your own future."

—*Roger Smith, American business executive*

After the hideous, expensive encounter with the shrink, I was more depressed than ever and didn't know where else to turn. I begrudgingly punched my zip code into that darn website Carol had sent me for the zillionth time. A directory of top local endocrinologists popped up on the screen. As I looked the list over, one name in particular leapt out at me. I didn't know why, but somewhere in the back of my mind I must have heard about him. I quickly dialed his number and found out he was booking appointments more than six weeks in advance. I picked the first date available and pleaded for an earlier cancellation. And that's how Dr. Mark Stolar of Northwestern Internists, Ltd., from Chicago's Northwestern Hospital, sailed into my life.

During the six weeks it took to get in to see Dr. Stolar, I knew I had to do *something* about my weight, so a friend suggested my husband and I give the Atkins Diet a go. He and I had always had pretty good results with following that low-carb diet in the past.

There are several key components that have to come together to successfully lose weight and keep it off forever. Picking the *right* diet* for you and really *sticking to it*, I've found, is one of the most crucial keys to true and everlasting weight loss and yet one of the most difficult. My husband also wanted to shed about twenty pounds (yeah, I know) and I appreciated his support for the tremendous amount that I needed to lose. It sure would make things a whole lot easier with both of us on the same diet page.

So, we did everything on that Atkins Diet—and I mean everything—by the book. He lost some of his weight, but I hardly lost a lousy ounce. It got to the point where you could threaten to flip me off a tall building with a single bounce before I'd consciously put a carb in my mouth. It was a matter of principle for me now. I was angry as hell. And dang it, I was bigger than this whole weight loss and food thing, wasn't I? I dug in my heels and made up my mind that I wouldn't cheat even for the winning Power Ball ticket. I was that determined.

I did have one last ace up my sleeve, however. Or so I thought. I had seen a news segment on TV about another form of gastric bypass, a less invasive procedure performed laparoscopically called the Lap-Band, which was being done locally at another university hospital. Naturally I went for the orientation. Still hoping for a miracle, I thought this was a much less drastic procedure and maybe it would be easier than the actual, hardcore gastric bypass.

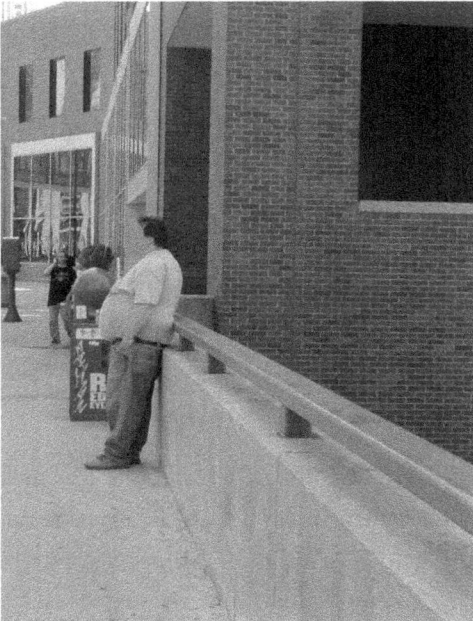

This time, the orientation was a group affair. The auditorium was packed to the rafters, overflowing to standing room only. On stage, the director of the program and the chief surgeon gave everyone interested in their Lap-Band procedure the low-down on this then-new surgical technique, cutting right to the chase. From there, they let you make up your own mind about whether or not you wanted to continue with the screening. I deliberated, but it was still apparent to me that in order to lose weight, it's up to you, the individual, to take the responsibility for controlling what you put in your mouth and moving your butt a whole lot more every day. *Same old, same old,* I thought. *Back to home plate.*

Crestfallen, I left the orientation and just kept up my Atkins Diet as best as I could until the six weeks passed and it was time for me to see Dr. Stolar. I did manage to lose about seventeen pounds on Atkins during those six weeks, squeaking my weight down nearer to the 300-pound threshold, but it was still nothing compared to what I really needed to lose and it was very s-l-o-w going.

Endocrinology and Carbohydrates

By the time I was finally admitted into Dr. Stolar's inner-sanctum exam room, I was bawling my eyes out. I was beyond despair and Stolar knew it. Between the sobs, snot, and tears, I blubbered my story to him: All the gory details about contemplating a gastric bypass, a Lap-Band procedure, and anything else I thought was "guaranteed" to spring me from being terminally stalled in weight-loss hell.

Without prejudging like all the rest of the medical professionals I had consulted and worked with Stolar who listened to every word I said very patiently and intently. He examined me, asked me lots of questions, and ordered extensive blood work. He told me he suspected I was probably hypothyroid and hyperinsulinemic (my pancreas creates too much insulin, which hampers the fat-burning process) and that I had an incredible sensitivity to carbohydrates from a lifetime of chronic overindulgence. *Hey, life's short, eat dessert first,* was always my motto. He wanted to see me back in a week, would have all the test results by then, and we'd go from there.

A week later he prescribed a natural thyroid medicine to help jolt that area into action, and he also put me on Glucophage twice a day. Glucophage is a diabetic medication Stolar felt would help regulate the insulin my pancreas overproduced.

I was not diabetic—not yet, thank God—but a lifetime of existing mostly on sweets and low-fat, white starchy carbs such as pasta, breads, rice, cereals, sweets and the like had sure taken its toll. As I now understand it, when I ate one Krispy Kreme donut, for instance, my pancreas would think I'd eaten about three or four and would push out enough insulin to compensate. The more white starch and sugar a person eats, the more insulin the pancreas produces.

"And what is insulin?" Dr. Stolar cheerfully quizzed.

I shrugged my shoulders and raised my eyebrows in a your-guess-is-as-good-as-mine kind of way. Hardly able to contain himself, he exclaimed, "It's the fat hormone, my dear. Why, insulin's the fat hormone! No wonder you've had problems controlling your weight your whole life."

A special thank-you to all my former doctors, registered nutritionists, dieticians, and shrinks, for believing in only *one* way to lose weight—their way, along with our wise and wonderful government's way: by eating low fat, even when it wasn't the right way for me and others like me. Your diet dogma was, and still is, severely outdated, so thanks for your professional opinions and alternatives, for not offering me a choice, and for not helping me find out what worked for my body and what didn't. I totally had to find out for myself.

In disbelief I told Dr. Stolar the same thing I'd told my friend, Carol, about every fat person in the universe just waiting to hear that it's not them—it's not their fault. It's "their system,"—their hormones—that are out of whack and keeping them fat.

Dr. Stolar then began to convince me to give him two years. "Just two years," he urged, "before you do anything rash, like go under the knife to lose weight." That's how sure he was of himself, his findings, and his ability to help me. He felt that by adjusting the two meds he prescribed for me, he would be able to regulate my system into being more efficient at controlling my insulin. This would in turn help me begin to burn calories, lose weight, and then maintain my lower weight and better health over the long haul.

Two years seemed like an eternity right then, but what did I have to lose? Only 130-150 pounds. Skepticism ruled me that day and I reluctantly nodded in agreement to give his method a try.

Since I was already familiar with the Atkins Diet and had more success on it than anything else thus far, Dr. Stolar okayed the plan with a few exceptions: "Eat low fat, also," he cautioned, "because you can develop a 'fat tooth' just like you can develop a 'sweet tooth.' And eat several servings of low-glycemic vegetables and at least one or two low-glycemic fruits a day." All this was easy enough to adjust to, so I agreed to give the whole process an honest try.

Once again, that strange calmness settled over me as I left Dr. Stolar's office and for a change, I wasn't in such a huge hurry. I was hopeful and relieved. I had a new direction and now needed to form a better, more precise plan of attack, the one that would work this time.

I have found, after all these years, the way to true and everlasting weight loss that finally works for me and others just like me—maybe just like you, too. I walk the walk and I walk the talk. "You are a do-er, a tell-er and a be-er," my favorite doctor proudly says of me, and with his, my husband's, and my two little dogs' help, I did it. I did it the old-fashioned way, taking my journey step by step, pound by pound, mile by mile, one foot in front of the other until I eventually reached where I needed to go.

I also called upon a higher power to help me spiritually and mentally. Using daily meditation to cultivate a stronger mind and spirit helped me develop a healthier, lighter, more alive body and lifestyle.

*As with any new diet and fitness plan, be sure to check with your physician before you begin.

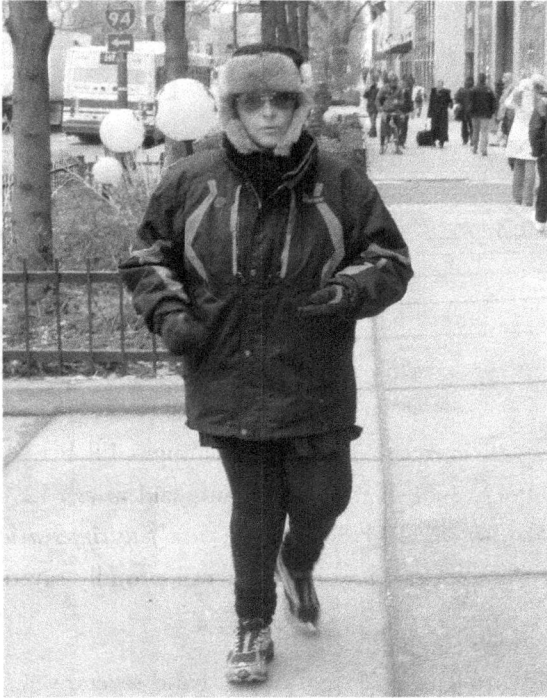

Don't you dare use the weather as an excuse
for not taking that cardio walk today.
Suck it up. Dress for it. Get 'er done!

Chapter 3

How Exercise Changed My Life

"First say to yourself what you would be, and then do what you have to do."

—*Epictetus, Greek philosopher*

How often do you exercise? Not nearly enough, I'll bet. According to a recent media survey, 35% of the respondents said *rarely*, 12% owned up to only a *few times a month*, 33% admitted to a *few times a week*, and only 20% said that they did daily workouts. I can proudly say that I'm in the daily 20%.

Before my knee problems really got out of hand several years ago, I shaved off 150 pounds strictly by walking five to eight miles a day—with a disability—and by following a healthy, effective low-carb diet. Now, after two knee replacements in the past few years, I'm eager to get my mileage back up before the snow flies because I know how good daily walking is for me.

Even though I currently cross-train every day, I manage to get in a minimum of an hour of cardio, regardless. I row for twenty minutes, then do twenty minutes on the Nu-Step—an awesome, non-weight-bearing recumbent climber. Then, after that, a minimum of twenty minutes on the Woodway Treadmill—a serious training treadmill all my marathon-running friends use for training indoors. The rubber-slatted bed keeps your back, hips, knees, ankles, feet, and legs from hurting.

If Not Now, When?

There's no time like the present to make it a goal to increase your walking stamina. I'm working on mine so that I can get back to walking five to eight miles a day. There's nothing, nothing, nothing that has ever helped me boil all my unhealthy weight off and keep it off like daily walking.

Speaking from over fifty years of up close and personal experience in the "Chronically Obese Diet and Fitness Wars," I do know that no matter what some of the media experts say, your weight isn't budging without a serious *daily* cardio workout—even with a good, healthy diet—so you'd better get busy or you'll never be Speedo worthy—ever.

I'm not telling you that you won't lose at least *some* weight by dieting alone, but not nearly enough. The first year of this last diet, I lost only forty pounds. Nothing to sniff at, I know, but I never realized how incredibly important daily exercise really is until I began to develop the habit for myself. Now, you can't shut me up about it!

I guess what I'm saying is once it was pointed out to me that I "played at working out," and once I saw what daily cardio did for a friend's husband, who lost the same amount of weight as I did but in a much shorter time frame, I kicked my cardio into high gear, making it my top priority every single day. And I know it will help you, too.

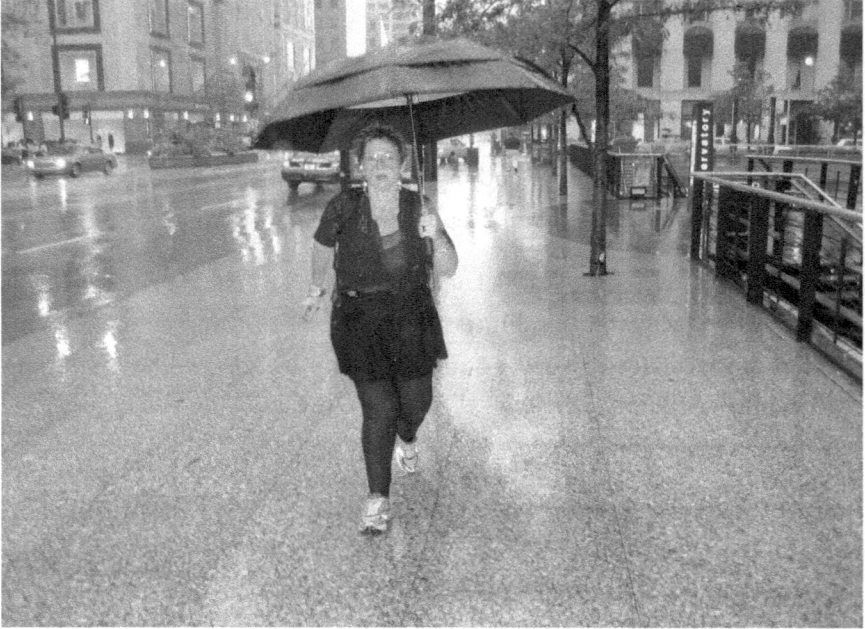

Walking 35,000 Miles in Ten Years

And that's exactly how I managed to walk over 35,000 miles—all the way around the Earth at the equator and then some—since January 1, 2003, leaving 150 pounds in my wake. And I'm ready to tackle the streets, once again, but this time, I'm giving myself several weeks to get my mileage tuned back up to my normal five to eight miles a day.

And you don't have to go out and kill yourself exercising eight hours a day, every day, like you're on "The Biggest Loser," either.

Weight loss and daily cardio aren't as difficult as they make it look on TV. Plain, old fitness walking did it for me—that, and cutting the white starch and sugar carbs from my diet. Each component continues to help me keep the weight off into my tenth year now and, hopefully, forever.

First, say to yourself what you have to say about the physical state you're in, then do what you have to do to get where you need to be health and fitness-wise. Begin right now—for the health of it.

Chapter 4

Never, Never, Ever Give Up

"Our greatest glory is not in never failing but in rising up every time we fail."

—Ralph Waldo Emerson
American poet and essayist

Thank God, the 4th of July is over until next year. It was a marathon-eating weekend for me and (it seemed) everyone around me—almost like my old, fat days. And, yes, even Laura, the "Low-Carb Diet Diva" slips off her scale every once in a while; no one's perfect. It's all a carb-coma blur …

Make no mistake - I do practice what I preach. I was back on my scale first thing this morning and wore that fabulous, new Woodway treadmill I'm so in love with at the club to an absolute frazzle. The treadmill, combined with all of the additional walking I did over the last few days, helped keep me from packing on the post-holiday pounds. Whew. Managed to dodge that one, but how about you?

Holiday Hangover

To give you an idea about this particular holiday, I went to an incredible party that Friday night and the food was, let me just say, *abundanza*. Then Saturday started off with a bang; I was invited on a wonderful walking food tour of downtown Chicago. Thank my lucky stars that we were walking in between each and every one of the food venues on the trip. I logged something like 5,183 steps, or two and a half miles in three hours. Our food guide, John, absolutely couldn't believe we walked that far. Nowhere near enough steps to make up for the carbs ingested, but wisely, I cut them everywhere I could, only eating big bites, half portions, doing whatever it took to lessen the overproduction of insulin's impact.

Saturday night found me on a private yacht cruising up and down the lakefront for Chicago's famous July 4th fireworks display—need I say more? I don't know if my stomach or my conscience got the better of me first, but much to my dismay, the funnel cake at a local fair the next day promptly lost its allure and I couldn't eat my half of the thing, even though I was dying to. And that was after eating almost a half-slab of ribs with slaw. Can you imagine? I'd fallen off the ole' proverbial wagon as nearly everyone else occasionally does, too. So it's time to climb back on.

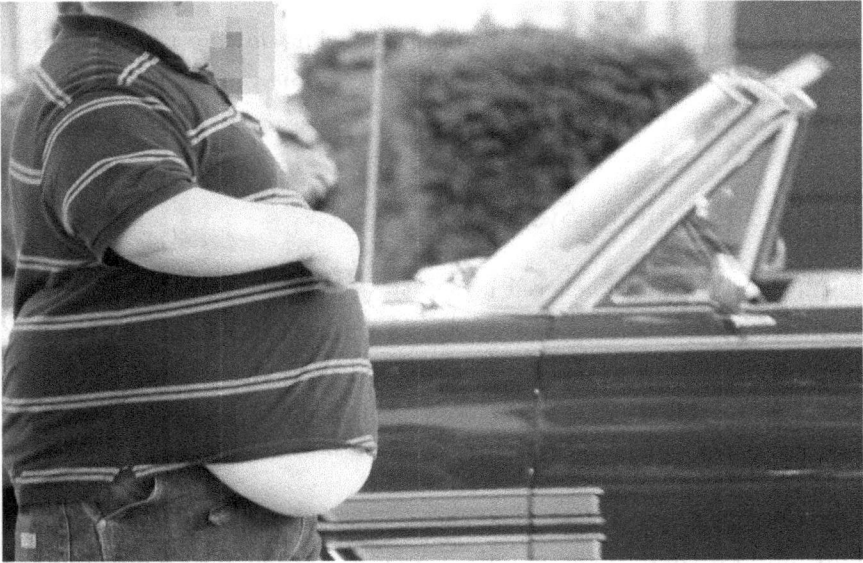

Getting Back On the Wagon

And sometimes it's the littlest things that set your motivation in motion. It can be something as small as a gal sitting with her back to me at the club's grille bar intently working on a Sudoku puzzle. What caught my gaze on the back of her tank top was so many "Nevers" written in a vertical row, spreading down her spine that my eyes crossed and I was unable to finish the count as I whizzed past.

A little later, I spotted the same woman working out in the cardio room and managed to tally that "Never" was listed nine times. I knew where her message was leading and gently touched her elbow to get her attention. I whispered as she turned toward me, "Thanks for reminding me that I have to keep on going and never, ever give up."

She gave me a warm, knowing smile and the thumbs-up as I turned to walk away. With that thought in mind, the last thing I wanted to do that day was my one-hour, post-holiday cardio walking—however, I knew I had to atone for my errant eating. You absolutely cannot exercise away a bad diet. But still …

My (and your) greatest glory is not in never failing on your previous weight loss and wellness attempts. It is rising up every time you think you've failed on your diet, health, and fitness plans and begin again, right where you are.

Find Your Support System

I'm lucky. I've always believed in myself—even now, when I feel insecure and have doubts. When I was younger, I was told that I was less by those who mattered most to me. It's hard *not* to believe them. Then I grew up. And I made sure I grew strong. And I made sure I always had the total support of myself, no matter what.

Over ten years ago, I discovered that I also had the total support of my husband in whatever I chose to do. I decided to really buckle down to lose 150 pounds, and he was right behind me from the start. Many people who come to me for motivational weight loss and fitness help don't have any support system at all. Instead, they've heard all about how fat they are, how they couldn't lose weight if their lives depended on it, how they can't do anything right, how worthless they are, how stupid and ugly they are, and a whole lot more. Life is tough enough without all that devious drama.

Obesity and poor health know no prejudice and have no bounds, but society has an ugly intolerance toward overweight people no matter how rich, famous, or powerful they are.

Sometimes the weight loss part is the least of it. Sometimes it's just proving to yourself that you can do something, anything, that's positive and supportive for you. Begin now to prove to yourself that you're stronger than those who say you can't; stronger than any foods that are keeping you fat; and stronger than being lazy and not getting out to exercise daily.

And never, never, ever give up.

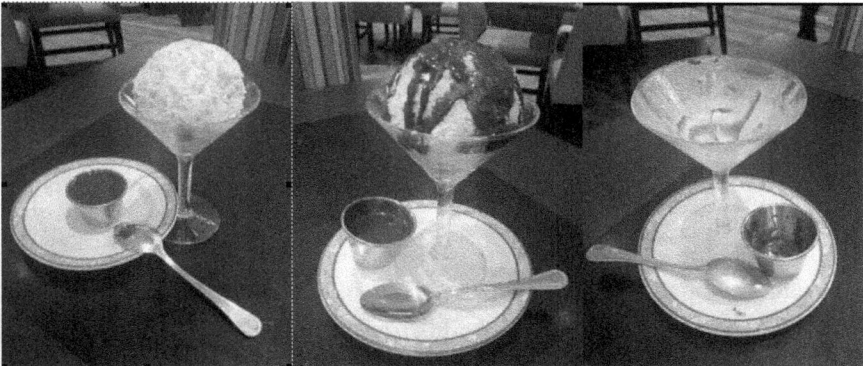

Sweet Tooth Extraction

If you're not careful, before you know it you could very easily snuggle into that horrid sugar addiction just like old times and far exceed your thirty-five grams of carbs a day. That's when you know you're headed for trouble.

When you're addicted to sugar and carbs as I am, you are addicted—period. It doesn't matter if you binge and eat the whole box of Dove milk chocolates or eat only thirty-five grams of chocolate carbs everyday … the addiction remains. So, in self-defense, I recently went to see Chicago's Dr. Elly Laser, Ph.D., who specializes in hypnotherapy. One of her specialties is what she calls the "Sweet Tooth Extraction." If there ever was a girl in need of having her sweet tooth extracted, it would be me.

This was the first time Elly hypnotized me and she said I was a hypnotherapist's dream because I slip into the hypnotic state very easily. While I like to be in control of my situation as much as I can, I excel when it comes to meditation and concentration, so being a great candidate for "Sweet Tooth Extraction" by hypnosis was not surprising for me. I hoped, anyway. I'm proud to report a couple months out that I lost a few more pounds, which my crazy chocolate addiction had kept on my frame and I feel even better for it.

And I didn't go out of my way to "test it out" like Elly warned me *not* to do. You have to build up that resolve while breaking your addiction. Both work hand in hand, and the Sweet Tooth Extraction hypnotherapy technique works like a charm—when you want it to. Like everything else in life that needs conquering or correcting or kicking, you gotta wanna. I wanna kick my chocolate habit bad enough that the process works for me, as long as I follow it. Sure, I can override it, but why, in heaven's name, would I when I've come this far?

How about you? How badly do you want to be more healthy and fit? Bad enough to kick your favorite food addiction to the curb by Committing To Get Fit with me once and for all?

Chapter 5

The Top Ten Excuses Why People Don't Go on Diets and Can't Lose Weight

"The human mind is like an umbrella, it performs best when open."

—*Anonymous*

When I say "people" here, I also mean myself; I was just as guilty as the next gal or guy when it came to finding excuses not to change. You have to make your new diet/eating plan and daily cardio routine your forever lifestyle so you don't regain lost weight. Period. There is no other way. See if you recognize yourself in any of the following statements.

1. I don't have the time to _____ (fill in the blank with shop, cook, or eat healthy; walk or exercise; do something about my weight or lifestyle because I work too much and I'm too tired.) You get the idea …

2. I hate exercising. It's too hard and boring. I'm too damn lazy. I can't do it. There's no facility near my house or office. I don't have the equipment or the clothes. I'm too out of shape to exercise in front of other people. I'm too out of shape to exercise at all. It hurts me to walk or do any kind of physical activity right now.

3. I'm looking for a quick fix. I want someone else to do it for me. Lemme take a pill. Gimme a gastric bypass or Lap-Band. (*Note:* Americans want it all now and we want it fast! Ain't gonna happen

by accident. Improved health and fitness take effort combined with daily diligence.)

4. I can't give up my _____ (fill in the blank with glass of wine with dinner, bread, chocolate, potatoes, bananas, oatmeal, rice, tortillas, beer, soda, popcorn, or whatever.) What might you refuse to give up in your pursuit of better health and fitness for life?

5. It's too painful to exercise; I have a sharp pain in my this, my that, and my other thing. I just can't walk. (See #2.) What if you started slowly, a little at a time, but did it every single day? There is no other way, no matter what anyone says, to get your unhealthy, unwanted, excess weight off other than with *daily* cardio and a good, healthy, effective diet, preferably one low in white starch and sugar carbs.

6. My _____ (fill in the blank with husband, kids, sister, brother, mother, father, lover, boss, coworkers, neighbors, friends, etc.) drive me nuts. It's all the stress of having to take care of everyone else first. I guess I'm just a stress eater. (Answer me this: What exactly *is* a stress eater? In my humble opinion, there is no such thing. I'll prove it to you—because when all else fails we eat better than anything else we do. Our eating technique is flawless; it's the one and only thing we can do and *not* be criticized for. Tell me I'm wrong. What else do you do that's THAT flawless?)

7. Why should I deprive myself? I work hard, I deserve to eat whatever I want. I don't want to go without ever eating my favorite foods again. No one's gonna tell me what to eat. I hate restrictions. I hate weighing and measuring food. It's boring to eat the same things all the time. I hate to count carbs or calories or anything.

8. I'm not *that* fat. A lot of people are in major denial about how fat and unhealthy they and their kids really are. They think, *I'm not plus-size; I don't shop in those stores or those departments. So what if I need a wheelchair to get around? My husband, lover, significant other,*

doesn't think I'm fat and likes me exactly the way I am. (Yeah, fat, frumpy, dumpy, outta shape, and "safe.")

9. I don't want to put forth the effort because the results are always the same. I eat all the right foods but still gain the weight back. Every time I go on a diet, I do really well, but the second I go off of it, I gain weight.

10. Are you afraid of alienating your husband, wife, kids, sister, best friend, lover, mother, father, significant other, etc., by becoming thinner and more beautiful? The fact is that most people are too comfortable in their ruts, no matter how much they complain and say they want to change. They just don't want to be healthier bad enough.

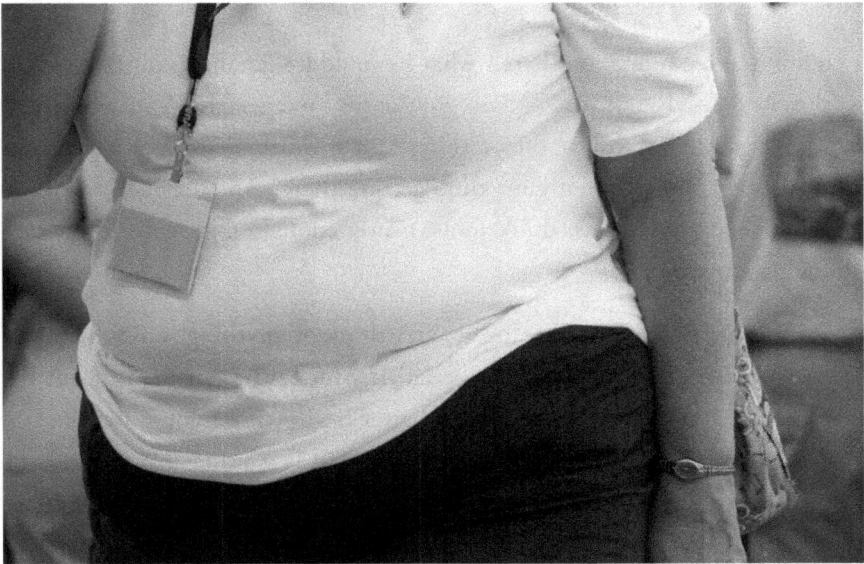

Have the Courage to Follow Your Heart

At just forty-eight years of age, Steve Jobs was diagnosed with pancreatic cancer. Two years later, on June 12, 2005, he gave the commencement speech at Stanford University. I am profoundly touched and motivated by what he had to say and know you will be, too. The following is a relevant excerpt from that speech.

"No one wants to die. Even people who want to go to heaven don't want to die to get there. And yet, death is the destination we all share. No one has ever escaped it. And that is as it should be. Because death is likely the single best invention of life. It's life's change agent. It clears out the old to make way for the new.

Your time is limited, so don't waste it living someone else's life. Don't be trapped by dogma, which is living with the results of other people's thinking. Don't let the noise of others' opinions drown out your own inner voice. And most important, have the courage to follow your own heart and intuition; they somehow already know what you truly want to become. Everything else is secondary."

I couldn't agree more, and here's what I can add: Certainly you don't want to die. And surely not just because you're way overweight. You will get to heaven regardless if you're fat or thin. And if death is the destination we truly all share, why hasten your time getting there? And all because you're lazy, eat the wrong foods, don't move nearly enough, and really don't care enough about yourself.

Obesity is life's change agent, too. I can't think of anything in my life more uncomfortable than how it felt to be fat. If you really want to clear out the old and make way for the new, you'd better begin with a good diet, health, and fitness plan right away, because a new you is waiting just around the next corner. Your weight and lack of fitness limit your time here more than you can ever imagine. Everyone thinks it won't happen to him or her, but just look around you to see how close to home the realities of obesity really hit.

And since your time here is so limited because of your weight and lack of fitness, there is no time like the present to get started on your way to improved wellness. Choose your diet, health, and fitness plans wisely. Do not be trapped by the same old, same old diet dogma of the past, no matter who it's from. Most just advocate outdated diets that never worked for you or me, either. No one's diet works for everyone.

Stop living with the results of other people's thinking. Pick a diet that's worked the best for you in the past and get on it right now, today. Then go to your doctor to let him or her know what you're up to. Open your mind and seek out new motivational methods to help you develop your new lifestyle, health, and fitness plans for a new, improved, better-than-ever you from this day forward. Don't let the noise of other's opinions drown out your own inner voice. Know that you *can* do it—whatever you set your mind to.

Just because you're overweight doesn't mean you're not a terrific, smart, beautiful person. Just think of how much better you'll be when you lose all your unhealthy, unwanted weight once and for all. And most importantly, I sincerely hope you have the courage to follow your own heart and intuition, because they do somehow already know what you truly want to become. It's never too late. The rest is up to you to figure out by working at it every day. Everything else—next to better health and fitness—truly is secondary.

No more excuses.

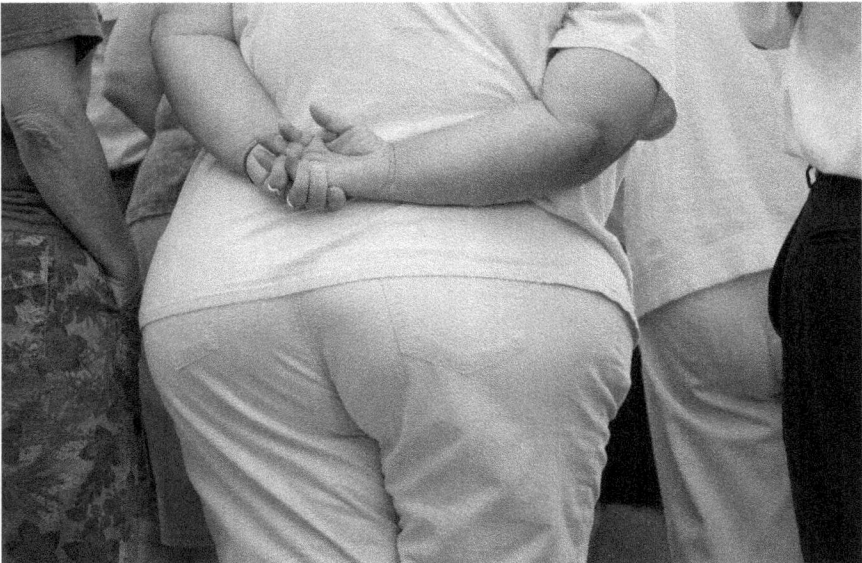

Part Two

The Politics and Science Behind Weight Loss

Chapter 6

How the Medical and Media Industries Keep Us Fat by Fueling the National Obesity Epidemic

"Whenever a doctor cannot do good, he must be kept from doing harm."

—Hippocrates, ancient Greek physician

Did You Know?

- National statistics tell us that over 50% of our population is obese. What percentage of those people will have their first heart attack within the year?

- Obesity is the second leading cause of unnecessary deaths.

- Obesity is a chronic disease with strong family components. For children, obesity could mean a lifetime of ridicule, medical problems, and worse.

- Obesity increases one's risk of developing conditions such as high blood pressure, Type 2 diabetes, heart disease, stroke, gallbladder disease, arthritis, and cancer of the breast, prostate, and colon.

- Environment and lack of physical activity, combined with high-calorie, high-carb, low-cost, low-quality foods, fosters the tendency toward obesity.

- Weight loss of as little as 10% of a person's body weight can begin to improve one's health.

- The National Institutes of Health (NIH) spends less than 1% of its annual budget on obesity research. Health insurance providers rarely pay for treatment of obesity, despite its serious effects on health. Promoters of fad diets, quick fixes, and junk food, on the other hand, spend millions on advertising.

- Obese people are frequent victims of employment and other forms of discrimination and are penalized for their condition, despite many federal and state laws and policies. Mistreatment of obese people is widespread and often considered socially acceptable in many circles.

- Obesity in women is one of the most serious public health threats in the country.

- The American Obesity Association says that 62% of women ages twenty to seventy-four are overweight, with 34% of them considered obese.

- According to The Cleveland Clinic, 80% of black women over the age of forty are overweight, and 53% of black women over the age of forty are obese.

- Heart disease, diabetes, high blood pressure, and certain cancers are now at epidemic proportions among women and are especially prevalent among black women.

It's no secret that obesity is an escalating epidemic in this country, but what would you say if I told you that much of it is due to medical, media, and economic politics, more than anything else? Most people continually struggle with their weight, especially those who are chronically obese and are on diet, health, and fitness plans that are wrong for them.

News Flash: There Is No One Diet or Health and Fitness Plan That Is Right for Everyone

Diet, nutrition, fitness, and medicine are like religions: There's the Food Group Pyramid faction, the low-fat fanatics, low-carb followers, Weight Watchers, Jenny Craigsters, Nutri-System supporters, and everyone else in between. Each one is a different school of nutritional thought, a different philosophy of medicine. And each one would have you believe their way is "The One and Only Way" for you, for everyone, to lose weight.

Stop looking for the magic bullet and start listening to someone who's actually lived it most of her life. I feel it's my mission, my duty, to help all those who wrestle with their weight the same way I did because of big business, politics, and medical and media malpractice.

In my humble opinion and those of a lot of other people, the media, big food, big pharma, and medical industries often put their own agendas first. When someone's views do not fit in with theirs and/or those of their "experts," the message doesn't get heard.

Given the availability in their areas and at their grocery stores, I believe if people made the right choices to buy fresh, lean beef, chicken and low-glycemic fruits and vegetables, *most* of the obesity problem would be gone within a year.

Their Profits Versus Our Health

All over the TV and radio, in newspapers and magazines, there's always some health, fitness, or nutritional expert telling us what to do and how to eat. But what do you think Big Sugar, Big Orange Juice/Big Every Juice, Big Cereal, and all the rest have in common? Economics, pure and simple. Most big businesses are more focused on profits at the expense of consumers' health—they're not concerned about your personal health, that's for sure.

For these industries, there are much lower profits in healthy food and in having a healthier America. The Food, Pharma, Media, and Medical industries all follow the money. When Big Pharma makes less, doctors make less, food producers and politicians all make less, so why would they want healthier consumers? Big Business always follows Big Profits. It's basic economics. Take away the high profit margins from sugar and carb-loaded food and snacks and watch what happens.

It's pretty amazing how they rely on the predictive buying habits of moms with kids, too. Commercials are mostly aimed at kids who pester the heck out of their parents to buy this stuff, just like toy commercials during the holidays. When are most of these food commercials broadcast? Certainly not during the day when the kids are at school - but from 6:00 to 8:00 p.m. and on weekend mornings during cartoons. It's no secret that highly focused marketing aimed at target buyers is how they do it.

Just look at food commercials, for instance - all sugar and carb loaded crap. Take a look at all the cereals and breakfast sweets for kids; everything that's advertised is all worthless, useless, carb-laden, destructive crap. There is no other word for it.

How many commercials do you see for skinless chicken breasts, broccoli, spinach, and lettuce made into healthy, yummy, low-carb salads? Or how about lettuce wraps at McDonalds instead of their thirty-two grams of carbs per tortilla wrap? Nope. Each and every one of the restaurant commercials are mostly high-carb, fast-food fare. (In all fairness, however, I *can* show anyone how to lose weight eating fast-food. I do eat it on occasion, but you have to know what to order to suit your healthier lifestyle.) The question is: how much do you really care about being healthier, thinner, and more fit? Enough to give up all the carby crap you're currently eating to maintain your heft?

Chapter 7

Certain Foods Really Are Addictive

"When everything seems like an uphill struggle, just think of the view from the top."

—*Unknown*

Many people claim that they don't have a problem with eating too much—they just have an addiction to certain foods. I did, too, until I got a grip and broke my addiction to white starch and sugar, then added an hour of daily cardio walking into my health and fitness mix.

I know only too well that each day is a battle for those who struggle with a food addiction that has plagued them for decades, as mine once did. We have become a nation of "sugar junkies." It's the white starch and sugar carbs that are making us fat and fueling our national obesity epidemic, not dietary fat.

Sugar Junkies

New research shows that some foods and other addictive substances have a lot in common. The experts claim that uncontrollable eating starts in childhood. I know my food addiction began way back then. My life's motto was always, "Life's short, eat dessert first." I did, and it showed.

It's said that many of us use food as a drug. We use it to self-medicate instead of dealing with life, but in the end, we're just plain old addicted to white starch and sugar carbs. Period. No question, food addiction is an affliction of the mind, body, and spirit, just like any other addiction.

However, what *your pancreas is really addicted to are white starchy, sugary carbs.*

I hate to sound like a broken CD here, but if you want to end your addiction to food, if you want to crush your cycle of compulsive overeating, then break your addiction to white starch and sugar carbs first. There is no other way. Seriously. Many health "experts" claim that you need to avoid certain foods (such as those high in fat) and eat only three measured meals a day—just enough food fuel to get through the day. This approach never worked for me. Until I broke my addiction to white starch and sugar carbs, my cycle of overeating continued to plague me all the way up to 317 pounds, not once, but three times in my life.

Well, no more. Food's hold on us is every bit as addictive as drugs or alcohol, and we evidence it on our bodies; we wear our addictions right up front for all to see, unlike most drug addicts and alcoholics.

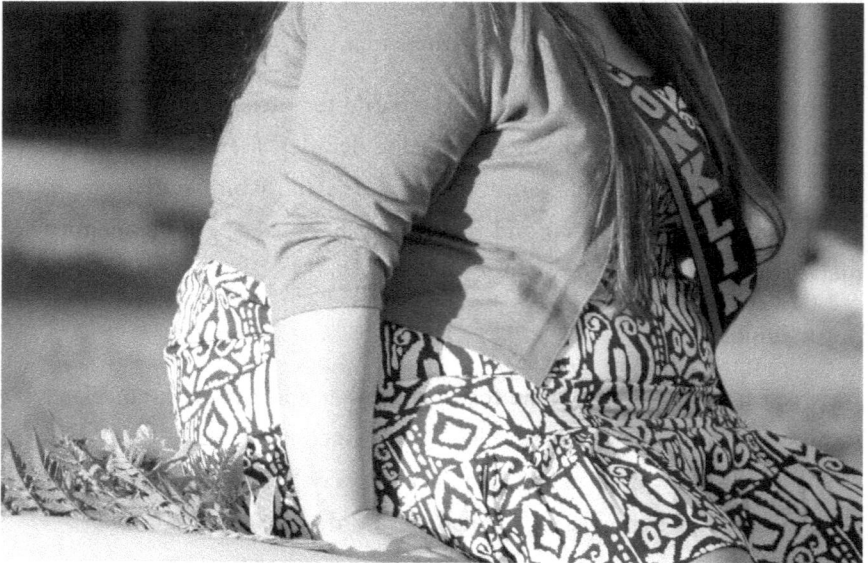

How Some Companies Keep You Eating … the Wrong Things

The following is an excerpt from "Here's Why Your Favorite Foods Are So Hard To Resist" by Renee Jacques, published in *The Huffington Post* on 10/16/2013.

(http://www.huffingtonpost.com/2013/10/16/junk-food_n_4043980.html?icid=maing-grid7%7Cmain5%7Cdl19%7Csec1_lnk2%26pLid%3D392383)

It's no secret: When you buy Doritos, you're going to finish the entire bag. There are countless reasons why people have so much trouble putting junky snacks down. And many of them are by design: Companies spend billions on marketing their products and conducting scientific studies to figure out how to engineer their foods to keep you eating.

Consider this: In a recent Connecticut College study, neuroscience students found that eating Oreos activated more neurons in the pleasure centers of rats' brains than did consuming cocaine or morphine.

And Michael Moss, *New York Times* writer and author of *Sugar, Fat, Salt*, recently wrote about ten components added to Doritos that make them extremely tasty and difficult to resist. Unsurprisingly, salt and sugar were major ingredients. In fact, the salty additives in Doritos give them a "flavor burst." That "burst" dissolves in your saliva, sending signals to the pleasure centers of your brain, explained Moss.

Do these foods sound "addicting" to you? Marion Nestle, professor of nutrition, food studies, and public health at New York University, and author of many books on nutrition, says there should be a distinction between having a strong desire for food and being addicted to it.

"I think of the word as meaning a physical dependence. We physically depend on food in general, but never on one food in particular," Nestle tells HuffPost. "Food companies create food products that people want to eat. Is wanting the same as addiction? I don't think so but there's evidence that foods trigger the same neurological pleasure centers as do addictive drugs, alcohol, and cigarettes, but not nearly to the same extent."

Read on to discover exactly how some of your favorite foods may be keeping you coming back for more.

You love pastries because they're packed with carbs. Lots of starchy foods contain complex carbs that your body breaks down into simple sugars. A study conducted on mice in 2012 found that *foods high in carbs, fats, and sugar can actually change the brain.* The researchers at the University of Montreal discovered that after being exposed to diets with high levels of fat and sugar, mice revealed withdrawal symptoms of depression and a greater sensitivity to stressful situations. They also had higher levels of the CREB molecule, which is known to play a role in dopamine production.

Much of this is still emerging science, and it's impossible to say that eating lots of sugar will necessarily make anyone feel happier, but humans are naturally drawn to sugary high-carb foods.

"We evolved to love the taste of sugars as an infant survival mechanism," says Nestle. "The brain needs sugar to function and carbohydrates are the most efficient source of it."

You love Cheetos because they literally melt in your mouth. How fast can you eat a bag of Cheetos? Probably pretty quickly. That's because the manufacturers of the puffed corn product have mastered the art of "vanishing caloric density." The Cheeto is extremely light and fluffy, therefore making it easy to rapidly melt in your mouth. Moss discovered that this junk food ploy tricks your brain into thinking you're not eating as many calories, so "you just keep eating it forever."

You love Fruit Loops, popsicles, and gummy bears because they are bright and colorful.

Now, of course, that's not the only reason why you love these tasty foods, but their vibrant coloring has been known to play a part. Food companies add color to their products to make them more appealing. Dr. Linda M. Katz, Chief Medical Officer for the Food and Drug Administration's (FDA) Center for Food Safety and Applied Nutrition, reports that color additives are incorporated into foods to "enhance colors that occur naturally" and to "provide color to colorless and 'fun' foods" (like popsicles and soda).

"That's what food companies do to sell foods," says Nestle. "That's their business. People don't like eating grey foods."

You love canned sauces because most contain excessive sugar. When we think of satisfying snack foods, tomato sauce isn't really on the list. But that doesn't mean it's free of the additives that make more typical junk foods more appealing. If you look at the ingredients list on a can of Prego tomato sauce, for example, the second ingredient after tomatoes is sugar, one of the three addictive components of fast food, according to Moss. The *New York Times* reports that just a half-cup of Prego traditional sauce has about two tablespoons of sugar. That's the same amount of sugar as in two large Oreos. Nestle says the added sugar in canned tomato sauces "makes them taste better and covers up the off, metallic taste from the canning process."

But before you head to the kitchen to make your own, note that sugar can be found in canned tomatoes—a common ingredient in homemade sauce—in the form of high-fructose corn syrup. If you're craving tomato sauce, you're better off avoiding any kind of tomato product that comes in a can.

You love candy because your body has not adapted to its intense flavor. There are a bunch of reasons why you can't resist munching on your kid's Halloween candy loot, but you can blame *part* of it on evolution. In an article on Prevention.com, Ashley Gearhardt, Ph.D., assistant professor in the psychology department at the University of Michigan, explained that the human body has not yet evolved to handle the intense trio of sugar, fat, and salt that comes in candy bars. Gearheardt wrote that before processed food was developed, sugar was "found in fruit and guarded by stinging bees; salt was a simple garnish; and fat was a nutrient that had to be hunted or foraged." These tastes taken together are still very new to the human body. (End of excerpt)

No Easy Way Out

I always tell people that I still consider myself a recovering, chronically obese woman. Only now I'm in remission, and just one really good hot-fudge brownie sundae away from 317 pounds and climbing, again. I've lived a lifetime like this, struggling just like a lot of you are right now, but I'm a healthier, happier, leaner, less encumbered, and more beautiful person these days. And I wouldn't go back to being that fat for all the tea in Taiwan.

A good, healthy, low-carb diet can and will help you finally stop struggling with your weight and achieve the same results I did—once and for all. Then you'll enjoy the improved fitness and wellness benefits of your dreams, all through healthy weight loss and maintenance.

In the end, ask yourself why we still have an obesity epidemic in this country with all these experts, gurus, and scientific smart guys running around hawking their "wares." Don't you think it's about time the American public was made aware of these diet dogma discrepancies and policies and realize that it's not necessarily the individual who's always at fault. Many people are simply on the wrong diet and fitness plan for them, despite what some of the experts say. For me and others like me, whose overproduction of insulin keeps them fat, the healthier choice is a diet low in white starch and sugar carbs.

And as soon as we, the consuming public, stop believing every "new-and-improved," "quick-and-easy" diet, health, and fitness gimmick and guru that comes down the pike, the better off we'll all be.

Do it for the health of it. If you're smart, you'll do it for your life because obesity is totally, unequivocally, and undeniably 100% preventable, which leads us into the next chapter, Obesity as a Disease?

Chapter 8

Obesity as a Disease?

"An ounce of prevention is worth a pound of cure."

—*Benjamin Franklin*
One of the Founding Fathers of the United States

How can something that's totally and unequivocally preventable be deemed a disease? I have read that disease is defined as a condition in humans, plants, or animals that results in pathological symptoms and recognizable signs often having a known cause but *is not the direct result of physical injury.* Chronic diseases are a serious problem in society.

Regardless of what the medical community says, it is my experience, opinion, and belief that obesity, even though it is currently a very serious societal problem, is not a disease because it is preventable. They might do it subconsciously, but people are choosing obesity by choosing to eat far too much of the wrong foods and refusing to move. We wear what we eat. No question.

Cancer, on the other hand, is definitely a disease. People do not choose to have cancer, even when exposing themselves to risks that increase the incidence of cancer, such as smoking.

I've lived a lifetime in chronic obesity's shoes and now I don't. I lost over 150 pounds on my own, and if I can do it, anyone can. That's why I do what I do: help motivate others to *Commit To Get Fit and Find the Secret to Their Own True and Everlasting Weight Loss* once and for all, just like I did.

These days, most people want it fast and they want it easy. Sadly, many people I meet or coach do not really want to make the effort to stop eating high-carb foods. The addiction to white sugar and starches and the refusal to do anything about it is what prevents people from losing their excess weight once and for all. No matter what they say, it is easier to have something or someone else do it for them. But just like everything in life, you have to work at it yourself.

The Body Mass Index (BMI) system is a standard, regulated approach of measuring obesity that is used by the medical community and the government. It is horribly antiquated and unrealistic for any person who is not a competitive athlete. BMI was developed in the mid-1800s and has numerous shortcomings, since it makes no account for muscle versus adipose (fat) tissues.

Because the BMI formula depends only upon weight and height, its assumptions about the distribution between lean mass and adipose tissue are inexact. Most professional athletes with high muscle volume are determined to be overweight or obese using BMI. In actuality, when using their percentage body fat as a measurement, they are in outstanding condition.

For example, according to this system, I am obese at 5'7" and 170 pounds, when I don't look that way at all. Your eyes, your scale, a mirror, and your clothes are better indicators of assessing your obesity situation. The current BMI system contributes to discouraging a great percentage of people when they lose weight, because according to their BMI, they are still obese.

When you know you are overweight, you either don't know what to do about it or are unwilling to make the necessary lifestyle changes to get rid of your unhealthy, unwanted weight. By proclaiming obesity a disease, the government and certification boards continue to dominate the health, diet, and fitness fields. The "approved and standardized" methods of dealing with obesity championed by doctors, board certified nutritionists, and dieticians are doomed to failure.

Why? The same old, same old, low-fat or calorie-counting diet dogmas, products, procedures, potions, and pills clearly are not working for enough people on a long-term basis. These methods may be what is keeping us in the middle of this proclaimed obesity epidemic. Unless our government and those in the medical and media professions open their minds to another way of addressing the obesity epidemic, nothing will change. Naming a condition (obesity) a disease makes it easier for doctors and other health and wellness professionals to get paid by insurance companies for treating something that's totally and unequivocally preventable.

Willpower and Healthy Eating

Recent studies say that one in three Americans are obese and that willpower isn't the only factor that comes into play when it comes to what we eat. But, if you ask me, developing willpower is one of the most crucial keys to true and everlasting weight loss. Once you break your addiction to white starch and sugar carbs and learn to improve your willpower, losing weight's actually not all that difficult.

I saw an interview with a woman who had a gastric bypass two years ago and lost 130 pounds, but was still struggling and still very fat. Her weight loss has slowed down because she eats way too many *high-glycemic* fruits, veggies, and "whole foods." Healthy foods? Not for her, nor others like her.

What exactly is healthy eating, anyway? It's not the same for every single person.

Plus, this gal isn't doing nearly enough daily cardio. If she were, her weight would literally fall off. And if you're overweight, neither are you.

Medicine is not an exact science, but please take a long, hard look at the white starch and sugars you eat and you'll find out why you have a food addition—and why you're fat.

True, none of us can live without food and we all have to find our own answers, but your white starch and sugar-carb addiction is the key. You know you're addicted when you have trouble pushing yourself away from the table and can't stop eating those white starchy and sugary foods that keep you hooked and compulsively craving more. If you're struggling with one diet after another, look at exactly what you're eating and drinking and *ditch the denial.*

Insulin is the fat hormone. *Too much insulin keeps you fat.* Just ask Chicago endocrinologist, Dr. Mark Stolar (Northwestern Internists, Ltd.), who listened to me, never prejudged because of my size, and showed me that those high-carb, high-glycemic foods were poisonous to my system. If you constantly struggle with one diet after another without successful, lasting weight loss, find a good endocrinologist of your own—one who understands the healthy, low-carb way to weight loss.

Education Is the Answer

People cannot be forced to eat healthier. But *healthy eating* can be redefined by considering the latest research on a healthy, low-carb way of life, instead of following the mantra of the lobbyists and big players in the food and drug industries, who are only interested in their own profits and not our health.

Educating people about how white starch and sugar carbs are making and keeping people obese is crucial to stemming the epidemic. Carbohydrates cause the body to overproduce insulin and keep people addicted, making them crave more and more of the same foods that keep them fat by fueling the addiction.

Look at school, hospital, assisted living, and other institutional food menus; it's all highly processed junk topped with juices and sodas. Throw in the obscene overuse of sodium that contributes to hypertension and these are the kinds of meals our insurance companies cover.

These foods are much more affordable (especially in large quantities) than fresher, healthier, whole food alternatives. Institutions must make profits to survive, so they are looking for low-cost options regardless of the potential health risks.

Then what do we do about the high-fructose corn syrup (HFCS) industry that the government subsidizes by giving farmers incentives, when HFCS is one of the most addictive sweetener substances on the market? Ever notice how, when you eat or drink something that you absolutely just cannot leave alone, something that keeps calling your name till you relent and eat or drink it till it's all gone? The culprit is always HFCS, trust me. Research the ingredients in the foods you buy and avoid anything with HFCS. Always read the labels!

Take Personal Responsibility

Ask yourself who has the largest vested interest in the obesity-as-a-disease issue. The government, medical, big pharma, and food industries would all lose money if obesity was successfully stemmed. There is no paranormal pill, procedure, or potion and no magic bullet for losing weight. It all comes down to taking personal responsibility and breaking the white starch and sugar-carb addiction. Period. You can easily find on the Internet the latest research about sugar addiction and what it does to the body. There are many books written on the subject as well.

And you cannot exercise away a bad diet, but a good, healthy, effective low-carb diet combined with daily cardio are two of the most crucial keys to true and everlasting weight loss. I'm living proof and so are hundreds of others who have successfully waged their own personal wars against their obesity struggles and won.

Classifying obesity as a disease does more harm than good because it removes the personal responsibility about their unhealthy conditions, so people can now blame being fat on "having a disease." You can prevent yourself from getting fat, but you cannot prevent yourself from getting most cancers. At least not yet.

Chapter 9

Carbohydrates and the Insulin Factor

"I was gaining weight very rapidly and read about the idea of restricting carbohydrates as an alternative to going hungry. I had a big appetite, so that was the only thing I would even consider."

—Dr. Robert Atkins, author and doctor

Dr. James R. Bailes is a pediatric endocrinologist who wrote the book, *No More Fat Kids: A Pediatrician's Guide For Safe and Effective Weight Loss.* He is another highly respected doctor in the endocrinology field who believes in the healthy low-carb way of weight loss and maintenance. A Clinical Associate Professor of Pediatrics at Marshall University School of Medicine in Huntington, WV, Dr. Bailes specializes in childhood obesity. He has developed an incredibly successful weight loss program for school-age children in which they lose weight without feeling hungry.

The program improves overall health, lipid profiles, and most importantly, self-esteem, and it has changed the lives of hundreds of children. His straightforward, practical, and easy-to-follow approach will change the lives of you and your child, too.

The following is contributed by Dr. James R. Bailes, from *No More Fat Kids: A Pediatrician's Guide for Safe and Effective Weight Loss,* 2006, Avant Garde Publishing.

This chapter is extremely important. At times, it is very technical. If you can understand this chapter, then you will understand the reason why this diet is successful, and it will allow you and your children to benefit just as many others have.

What is a carbohydrate? Basically, all foods can be broken down into several different components. First, we have the energy suppliers, carbohydrates, proteins, and fat. Food also consists of micronutrients—vitamins and minerals. All food also contains water. The term carbohydrate covers an immense variety of edible food. Breads, pasta, potatoes, fruits, refined sugar, flour, candy, many vegetables, and most junk foods are purely carbohydrates. All sugars, starches, and most fiber we eat are all carbohydrates. Varied as these foods may be in color, texture, taste, and nutrient content, the carbohydrates contained in most of them are quickly transformed by the body into one essential substance: glucose. Glucose is the main sugar in the blood and the body's basic fuel. For animals as well as humans, glucose provides the primary source of energy.

To most people, "sugar" means white table sugar (sucrose) made from sugar cane or beets. However, sugar comes in many other forms. In its pure form it has names such as fructose, dextrose (glucose), lactose, maltose, sorbitol, and xylose. Sugars may also be identified by their sources, such as honey, corn syrup, maple syrup, and molasses.

The sugars in fruits contain a combination of dextrose, fructose, and sucrose, which are all rapidly converted to glucose by the body. All sugars are essentially the same and none offer any significant nutritional advantage over another. That is, there is no difference between honey and a baked potato, a bowl of cereal or a candy bar, an orange, or a spoonful of table sugar. All of these carbohydrates are quickly converted into glucose, which is used in your body as energy, stored in your liver as glycogen, or stored as fat.

Am I saying that an apple is no better for you than a spoonful of sugar? No. An apple has many other ingredients that are good for you, such as fiber, vitamins, and minerals. An apple is going to help fill your stomach and satisfy your appetite because of the fiber. An apple also has water. However, as far as the sugar content goes, an apple is just like eating a spoonful of sugar plus the vitamins, minerals, fiber, and water.

What about complex carbohydrates? These must be okay, right? Complex carbohydrates are actually large chains of glucose or other simple sugars that are connected together. These so-called starches are found in many types of food including breads, potatoes, and many vegetables. Since your body primarily uses glucose as an energy source, these complex carbohydrates are broken down or digested into sugars (monosaccharides) that are easily converted to glucose.

This digestion begins in the mouth when the enzymes in saliva split these large polysaccharides into smaller and smaller pieces. The digestion continues in the stomach and the small intestine, where these simple sugars are absorbed. Complex carbohydrates must be broken down into simple sugars *before* they can be absorbed. Therefore, if we eat a baked potato, it is metabolized into thousands of simple sugars and then absorbed. It is really no different than eating a mouthful of pure sugar with added nutrients.

Complex carbohydrates also contain fiber that occurs in all plant foods. Fiber is a crucial item in the carbohydrate package and comes to us from such plant foods as whole grains, fruits, and vegetables. Insoluble fiber provides bulk in the intestine and helps regulate bowel movements. Due to our high consumption of refined white flour (which has less fiber than whole grain flour) and our preference for sugary foods over whole grains, fruits, and vegetables, fiber has decreased tremendously in the American diet.

Children in particular are vulnerable to these low-fiber diets, especially in regard to their bowel patterns. It has been well-documented that chronic constipation, which often results from decreased fiber intake, is the most common cause of abdominal pain in children. I see this at least once a week in my general pediatric practice. A child will come to me with severe intermittent crampy abdominal pain that is caused solely from constipation. A diet high in fiber can often prevent or treat this problem.

Since the majority of carbohydrates are broken down into glucose, why does it matter which carbohydrates you consume? Complex carbohydrates are better for us because they also contain many other things such as fiber, small amounts of protein, iron, calcium, and many other vitamins and minerals. *However, except for these vitamins, minerals, and fiber, complex carbohydrates should be thought of just like pure sugar.* Simple sugars on the other hand contain only carbohydrates without these added benefits. They are empty calories.

Insulin—Villain or Victim?

What about insulin? We've heard many things about insulin, both good and bad. Which are true? This insulin hormone is one of the most powerful and efficient substances that your body uses to control the use, distribution, and storage of energy. Insulin is a protein hormone that is produced in the pancreas by cells that are grouped together in what are called islets of Langerhans. These cells secrete insulin in response to how much glucose is absorbed in the small intestine. Insulin is essential for life. It is the key that allows glucose to enter the cells of the body and be used for energy. Without insulin, we would quickly waste away and perish. Just ask the teenager with Type I diabetes, who has been recently hospitalized for diabetic acidosis and almost died because of not taking his or her insulin.

Insulin historically has been associated with blood sugar. Insulin was first isolated from the pancreas in 1922 by Drs. Banting and Best. Almost overnight the outlook of the severely diabetic patient changed from rapid decline and death to that of a normal person. Insulin certainly has a profound effect on carbohydrate metabolism. In combination with glucagon, these two powerful hormones establish and maintain very stable blood glucose values. Insulin also has profound effects on fat metabolism. Insulin can direct protein metabolism and essentially control the production of glucose by converting amino acids (the building blocks of protein) into glucose.

What Happens After a Meal High in Carbohydrates?

As we have seen, carbohydrates are broken down into thousands of molecules of glucose that are quickly absorbed through our small intestines into our bloodstream. Our body then has the ability to monitor this rapid rise in blood sugar and quickly secretes insulin to counterbalance this. Our nervous system must be supplied with a consistent amount of fuel. Therefore, our bodies keep our blood glucose levels very steady, no matter what we eat. These values almost never get above 120 mg per deciliter or lower then seventy. They usually stay stable between ninety and 110. This is true whether we eat a meal that consists only of pure sugar, a meal loaded with complex carbohydrates, a meal consisting of only protein and fat, or when we have fasted for two or three days. Almost all of the cells in our body use glucose for energy.

It would seem reasonable to suppose that if we have more glucose in our bodies, we would have more energy and feel better. However, this is not the case. Our bodies are extremely efficient energy machines: only a small part of what we eat is actually used or needed by the muscles or other cells of the body for energy. If these energy-using cells do not need any extra energy, what happens to the majority of the glucose we ingest? Well, as the sugar in your blood rises, insulin rushes in and converts a portion of that glucose to another starch called glycogen. Glycogen is stored in the liver and can maintain our blood sugar values in the normal range for a few hours after a meal. This is why we do not have to eat continuously.

Glycogen can be quickly converted to glucose by the cells in the liver or muscles whenever glucose is not readily available in the bloodstream, which is one of the most important functions of insulin. It causes most of the glucose absorbed after a meal to be stored immediately in the form of glycogen. Then, between meals, when food is not available and the glucose concentration begins to fall, the liver glycogen is split back into glucose and released back into the bloodstream to keep the blood-glucose level from falling too low. Approximately 60% of the glucose absorbed after a meal is stored as glycogen.

What about the rest of the glucose? Where does it go? After the liver is filled with glycogen and can hold no more, then it changes its production and converts glucose into fatty acids. These fatty acids are then transported to the blood where they are taken to fat cells and then stored.

> *Herein lies the answer to why most low fat diets do not work: The extra glucose is converted to fat. Fat is our main storage area for energy. Most of our bodies have enough stored fat to be able to walk over 1,000 miles without ever having to eat a bite of food. Let me say this again, insulin promotes the production and storage of fat.*

Excess Carbs Turn into Fat

That's right, even without eating fat, our bodies produce fat. If our diet consisted totally of carbohydrates, protein, and a very small amount of the essential fat (linoleic acid), then we would still become overweight and over fat.

> *This explains what I have seen in my practice and why millions of people in the world have failed to lose weight on a low calorie, low fat diet. This dietary approach works for about one out of every twenty-five people. As previously noted, it worked for only a very small percentage of children that I had placed on a low-fat, low-calorie diet. However, as a physician, a low-fat dietary approach is what is drilled in our brains. This is what society faces daily: We're told we must eat low-fat foods in order to lose weight. It just doesn't work and now you know why.*

> *The moral of the story?*

> *As physicians, what might we assume when a patient placed on a low-fat, low-calorie diet returns for follow-up two months later and he has not lost weight but instead has gained three pounds? Of course,*

we'd assume that person has been noncompliant with our directions; certainly if he had been following our plan, he would have lost weight. We put the blame back on the patient or parent. We make them feel guilty and tell them to try harder. You can see where this leads. The patient quickly becomes frustrated, distrustful, and abandons the diet. He feels hopeless, depressed, and often resorts again to overeating. Increased fat, increased carbs and a vicious cycle resumes. It's time to break this cycle.

Let's get back to how insulin contributes to this cycle. As I mentioned earlier, insulin is an extremely efficient hormone and the master hormone of our metabolic system. Its most important function may be the control and maintenance of our blood sugar, but insulin performs a myriad of other activities. In the appropriate amount, insulin keeps the metabolic system running smoothly with everything in balance. However, in great excess it becomes a dangerous hormone wreaking havoc throughout the body.

Mountains of scientific studies (many of which are added weekly) implicate insulin as the primary cause or significant risk factor for high blood pressure, heart disease, arteriosclerosis, and high cholesterol. It has also been implicated as having a causative role in Type 2 diabetes. We can control our insulin secretion by controlling and changing our diet.

Insulin has several different effects that lead to excess fat storage. One is the simple fact that it increases the utilization of glucose by most of the body's tissues. This automatically decreases the utilization of fat. Insulin therefore acts as a "fat sparer," which is another reason it is hard to lose weight by following a low-fat, low-calorie diet. The majority of calories are obtained from carbohydrates, which stimulate insulin, which spares fat.

Life Without Insulin

When insulin is not present what happens in the body? In the absence of insulin, all of the effects of insulin-stimulating fat storage are reversed. Enzymes in the fat cells become strongly activated, causing a breakdown of stored triglycerides into free fatty acids. These fatty acids are the main energy supply for essentially all tissues of the body except the brain. (The brain does not need insulin to be able to utilize glucose). These fatty acids are also converted in the liver to ketone bodies, which is called ketosis. Ketone bodies are utilized as energy for many tissues in the body.

When insulin is not available to promote glucose entry into the fat cells, then fat storage is blocked. Therefore, *if you don't have excess insulin, you cannot become fat.* What about excess fat intake? If I cut out my carbs but eat a lot of fat, won't I still become overweight? The answer is no. *Insulin is the key hormone that drives fat storage.* It doesn't matter how much fat you eat, as long as you have a low amount of circulating insulin, you will not become fat. Now this is not to say that you can eat all the fat that you want. This phenomena only works if you are eating much fewer carbohydrates. If you continue to eat a lot of carbs and also eat more fat, then not only will you not lose weight, but you will gain weight even faster.

Let me tell you about Lisa, a fifteen-year-old patient of mine, who has had diabetes for eight years. She had been treated with insulin since her initial diagnosis when she was in the second grade. Unfortunately, juvenile diabetes is often very difficult to treat. We try to match her insulin amount with her food intake. Sometimes we are successful and other times not. If we give too little insulin, then blood sugars run too high, which can lead to numerous long-term complications. If we give too much insulin, then blood sugars often become too low (hypoglycemia).

Too much insulin also leads to excess weight gain. This is exactly what happened to Lisa; she began to gain weight too quickly just shortly after her initial diagnosis of juvenile diabetes. She continued to gain weight at a fairly rapid clip until puberty when she exploded with a forty pound weight gain in one year. She was thirteen years old and weighed 238 pounds.

As a result of her diabetes and her obesity, Lisa became depressed and almost suicidal. She decided that she needed to lose weight. However, she approached it in the wrong way by quitting her insulin altogether. Yes, she lost weight, but she almost died. Most of her weight loss was secondary to severe dehydration and muscle wasting. She quickly slipped into diabetic acidosis and suffered severe electrolyte abnormalities. Fortunately, Lisa made it to the hospital, where she was successfully treated with insulin and IV fluids before it was too late. I knew we needed to make some drastic changes in her insulin regimen to allow her to lose weight or she may not be so lucky next time.

Lisa had previously tried to lose weight by cutting back her calories and exercising more, which never seemed to work. We talked to Lisa about our weight-loss project and she decided to give it a try. I was a little hesitant at first. We had seen great results in children of all ages, but she was different. She had diabetes. She was at risk to suffer severe low blood sugar reactions if she didn't eat carbohydrates. I knew that most of her weight gain was from excess insulin, so if she didn't need this extra insulin, then hopefully she would lose weight.

We took a chance because she was at the end of her rope. It worked! We saw just as dramatic results as did our other children following our diet plan. She lost twenty-eight pounds in three months and continued to lose weight until she had reached her goal weight of 175 pounds. We did have to make some major changes in her insulin regimen. She required much less total insulin because her carbohydrate intake was much less. She felt better, and her attitude changed. Lisa is presently doing great. Her blood sugar values are the best they have ever been.

Chapter 10

How Safe Is the Atkins Diet Versus Other Diets?

Part 1: Laura's Experience

> *"What you get by achieving your goals is not as important as what you become by achieving your goals."*
>
> —*Goethe, 18th century German politician and author*

After living a lifetime in chronic obesity's shoes, I finally lost all of my unhealthy, unwanted weight on my own without any surgery or gimmicks. I can personally attest to the fact that the Atkins Nutritional Approach™ to weight loss is safe for most overweight and chronically obese people. It saved my life. I lost 150 pounds and still live the Atkins lifestyle during the week and save "cheat meals," not "cheat days," usually for Saturday nights. Sometimes Friday nights, too, depending upon what's going on socially. I'm going to show you how you can lose weight just like I did—without the constant struggle.

The biggest difference in my eating habits now is that I know where to draw the line when it comes to harmful, white, starchy, sugary carbs that I used to eat with total abandon, thinking I was eating "low-fat healthy." No more. Now I know better. And so will you when you finish reading this how-to book.

I have been following a modified form of the Atkins Nutritional Approach™ lifestyle eating plan since I began my personal weight-loss transformation project in late summer of 2002. It took me 2½ years to shed 130 pounds, and I continue to maintain my weight loss to this day.

In the summer of 2009, I had a total right knee replacement and managed to shed another twenty pounds during my six-month rehab simply by upping my daily cardio quotient from sixty to ninety minutes a day. I'm proud to say that I have absolutely no problem with my kidneys or any other organs in my body because of my lower-carb lifestyle, and all my critical cholesterol LDL, HDL, and other numbers are much lower as a result.

How to Stay on Track and Motivate Yourself

A calorie is a calorie is a calorie—except when it's a carbohydrate. It's not only consuming too many calories that makes us fat, it's also eating too many carbs, and not doing enough daily cardio. (But that's another story we'll discuss further on in this book.)

During my personal weight-loss transformation project, my endocrinologist-internist, Dr. Mark Stolar, saw me every few weeks at first, then every six weeks. As my weight loss progressed, I saw him about every three months. He kept close tabs on all my numbers by taking blood tests at every single visit. This is something I strongly suggest you do: get a good, thorough health screening from an endocrinologist who understands and believes in the healthy, low-carb way of weight loss. It does make a difference when you're both on the same wavelength with regard to diet dogma and daily cardio. Having the accountability factor of seeing your doctor and your motivational weight loss coach regularly really helps, too.

I had to be my own motivational coach. I had to figure things out on my own—what worked, what didn't. But, I was so highly motivated to get rid of my excess weight that I was delirious with joy just to see the scale going down almost daily, but surely weekly—even if sometimes it was only a quarter of a pound. I celebrated each and every ounce I lost and used the number I saw on my daily morning weigh-in as motivation throughout the rest of my day. And if it worked for me, it'll certainly work for you, too.

I'm absolutely convinced, without question, that people who constantly struggle with their weight are pretty much the same as me: extremely carb sensitive, insulin-resistant, hyperinsulinemic. For us, no matter how complex the carb, a very little goes a long, long way toward keeping us fat from the overproduction of insulin. I know I found out the hard way.

I don't even eat whole wheat bread, whole wheat pasta, brown rice, or even quinoa to this day. Yes, I'm *that* carb sensitive. And you might be the same, too.

Remember: You Wear What You Eat

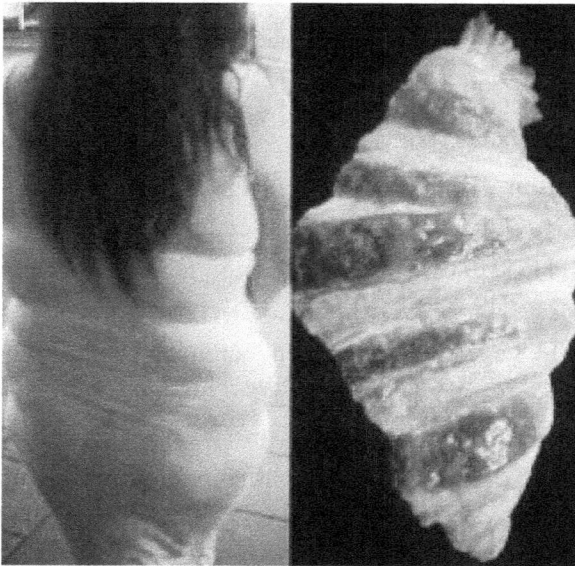

How do I know all this? Because I conducted my own personal research by tracking my weight, walking, weight training workouts, Pilates, and everything I ate on a daily basis. This enabled me to monitor my weight loss very closely and I knew when I didn't lose, it was due to what I was eating, period, because I certainly was getting in enough daily cardio by walking five to eight miles a day. I made sure of it.

Whole grains, whole wheat pasta and bread, oatmeal, brown rice, sweet potatoes, and the like do not mean enough to me anymore to sacrifice my weight loss just to "eat healthy," as some doctors, nutritionists, and TV weight-loss experts would have you believe. That stuff is not healthy for anyone who overproduces insulin like me. Yet, the experts don't ever tell you that, do they? And I'm living happily and healthily without ever eating any of these things again. Actually, I've lost my taste for them, almost entirely. Follow my advice and you will, too.

If someone would have told me this would happen to me at the beginning of this diet, I never, in a thousand years, would've believed them. But, it's true. Once you break that white starch and sugar addiction, and keep it broken, you're home free. It's when you start cheating here and there, when you think you can outsmart yourself, outfox your pancreas, and outwit your demon that you can get into trouble.

The more you cheat on your low-carb diet* (or any diet, for that matter) the less likely you are to have long-term success. First, get the weight off, then worry about maintaining and squeezing in a cheat meal here or there. By then, you'll know exactly what you can and cannot get away with.

I've Lived an Entire Lifetime Like This

Here's what some of my previous doctors, nutritionists, registered dieticians, shrinks, and trainers told me when I wasn't losing any weight on their program: "You're cheating." "You're not being honest about what you're eating." "You're not writing down everything you're eating every day in your food journal." Blah, blah, blah. Never once did any one of them question their professional methods and think maybe, just maybe, what they were prescribing possibly wasn't the right diet for me?

Never once did any one of them question themselves. Why should they? Weren't they the "medical professionals," after all? Guess what? Now I know better. Now I know it was never me. It was them all along. Each and every one of them had me on the wrong diet, health, and fitness plan for me.

And if, in your heart of hearts, you know you're following your physician's weight-loss plan at least 95% of the time, just like I was, and you're not enjoying enough (or any) positive weight loss results, you need a change. Find another doctor. You're obviously different than the rest of their clientele and need to find another way. You need to work with someone who can help you find the diet that's just the right one for you.

I constantly struggled and beat myself up over one diet failure after another—for a lifetime. And if you ask me, I wouldn't go back to the way I was then for anything in the world. Being this much healthier, thinner, and lighter on my feet, legs, and spine is way more fun than being chronically obese. I have never looked or felt better and younger.

I will also tell you that *it's way more difficult to stay fat, maintaining and sustaining that heft, than it is to just get the weight off and keep it off once and for all.*

Additionally, I also felt the South Beach Diet was too convoluted for me, personally. I'm way too hyperinsulinemic to eat even the slightest hint of harmful (or even complex) carbs, as I've discussed earlier. The carbs in rice and whole grains do the same thing to me that white starch and sugar do: they make me overproduce insulin, thereby retarding my weight loss, keeping me addicted—and fat.

How do I know this for sure? I tested it myself time after time after time. I weighed myself every single day and kept a strict log of as much of the data as I could.

Not everyone can eat those "healthy" foods and still lose and maintain their weight. Sorry, all you doctors, health care professionals, and hard-core scientists out there, who still believe that dietary fat is the artery-clogging villain. Quite often, it's the diet you have your patient or client on that's the real culprit leading to failure, not the person in your care.

Change Your Diet, Change Your Result; Change Your Result, Change Your Life

One thing I like about the Atkins no-nonsense approach to the induction phase of their diet is that you can do the quick start by totally removing all harmful carbs for just three days. And you can do anything for three days, can't you? It's not an eternity. Besides, there's nothing I like better than cutting right to the chase to get things rolling. Life's too short to mess around.

South Beach's two-week induction seems like forever when you're desperate to see some results—and that's a bit too long for me to work at inducting myself into anything, let alone a new diet and weaning off white starch and sugar carbs.

Please consult the latest version of *The New Atkins for a New You* for a more detailed explanation of how the diet really works and the effect it's going to have on your body, so you understand and appreciate what's happening to you every step of the way.

All this info is my impression based on my experience and a lifetime of personal research (see the Medical Resources section at the end of this book). All I can say is, a modified, lower-fat Atkins Diet worked for me like nothing else ever before in my life, and continues to help me keep my weight off much more easily than I ever thought possible.

Then there's the all-important daily cardio factor that figures into true and everlasting weight loss, but we'll get into that part of the fitness equation later in the book.

Part 2: Atkins Nutritional Approach™

Contributed by Colette Heimowitz, Vice President, Atkins Nutritionals

The Atkins Diet, also known as the Atkins Nutritional Approach™, should not be followed as a quick way to shed a few pounds. The approach is meant for those that seek a lifestyle change that involves better eating habits, ultimately leading to better health and a sense of well-being.

Scientific research has consistently and increasingly demonstrated the benefits of a controlled-carbohydrate approach in the face of the standard American diet of white flour, sugar, and other junk foods. There has been more than forty years of independent research on ketogenic diets, thirty years of clinical experience at the Atkins center, and now over ten years of clinical trials looking specifically at the Atkins protocol, which have demonstrated safety. These studies were funded by prestigious institutions, such as the American Heart association, NIH, Veterans Administration, and teaching universities and hospitals, all of which demonstrated safety and efficacy. No other diet program has been studied so extensively. Duke University and John Hopkins Hospital now routinely use the Atkins Nutritional Approach™ in treating patients.

When you are following Atkins, there are several health benefits, the most important of which is stabilized blood sugar. For many obese individuals, eating excess amounts of carbs was the reason for their weight gain. Their blood sugar was constantly in flux, leaving them tired and shaky when it was low and *craving more carbs.*

Excessive carb consumption can also produce spikes in the production of insulin, a hormone which is responsible for transferring glucose from the blood to the cells for energy and the carbs that are not burned are stored as fat. Continued overproduction of insulin is not healthy and can lead to obesity and metabolic syndrome, which is the body becoming resistant to the effects of insulin, a precursor to diabetes, which often goes hand in hand with obesity and heart disease.

Trimming carbs can improve blood-sugar levels, perhaps even lessening the need for glucose-lowering medications for diabetics. A study published in the medical journal *Diabetes,* "Effect of a High-Protein, Low-Carbohydrate Diet on Blood Glucose Control in People with Type 2 Diabetes," comes to the conclusion that low-carbohydrate diets can dramatically "reduce the circulating glucose concentration in people with untreated Type 2 diabetes." The conclusion drawn by the study is "potentially, this could be a patient-empowering way to ameliorate hyperglycemia without pharmacological intervention."

Ultimately, after the adaptation phase, those following Atkins usually report high energy and clear thinking throughout the day. This is possible because their blood sugar has been stabilized; they're avoiding blood-sugar peaks and valleys throughout the day, putting an end to mood swings and periods of lethargy.

Those who experience high blood sugar due to insulin resistance may also have, or are likely to develop, high blood pressure. The Atkins approach is also useful in bringing this kind of high blood pressure down. Following Atkins will result in a loss of excess weight and a stabilized blood sugar, which are both factors that will assist in returning blood pressure to normal levels.

> *The Atkins Diet* has been associated with an increased risk for heart disease. Emerging research has contradicted this many times, though, including a study from the American Journal of Medicine. This study, comparing a low-carbohydrate with a low-fat diet approach, found that subjects at a high risk for coronary artery disease (CAD) who were following the low-carb approach had improvements in their good and bad cholesterol profiles, allowing them to decrease their risk of developing CAD.*

With its ability to help you lose weight, improve your lipid profile and blood pressure, increase your energy and reduce your risk of heart disease, diabetes, and many other life-threatening conditions, the Atkins Nutritional

Approach™ is indeed a healthier, more balanced way of eating and living. When an individual is following Atkins correctly, the amount of protein consumed is within the limits of safety.

There are also many digestive benefits that come with following Atkins. Because the Atkins Diet replaces highly refined, low-fiber carbohydrates with salad greens, fresh vegetables, low-sugar fruit, nuts, seeds, and eventually whole grains, fiber requirements can be easily met.

> *A misconception about the Atkins Diet is that it is low in fiber, when in fact, it includes lots of vegetables to replace processed foods which increases fiber intake. A high-fiber diet is indeed the best way to lower risk factors associated with the colon. Additionally, numerous scientific studies have confirmed that those eating a high-fiber diet have lower cholesterol levels and less incidence of heart disease than those on a low-fiber diet.*

On Atkins, one consumes 25% to a maximum of 30% of calories from protein, which is not considered high. Although excessive protein intake remains a health concern in individuals with preexisting renal disease, most literature lacks significant research demonstrating a link between protein intake and the initiation of progression of renal disease in healthy individuals.

A myriad of derivative low-carbohydrate programs have sprung up over the past few years all claiming to be "a new and improved" version of Atkins. But the truth is, there is little, if any, difference between them and Atkins—other than the fact that the Atkins Nutritional Approach™ has been scientifically validated as safe and effective in numerous studies, for up to two years in length, while the imitators remain untested. The wasted energy used to "spin" these programs as somehow better than Atkins should be put to better use in a discussion about the existing science, which can truly help us battle the epidemics of overweight and obesity.

The South Beach Diet* is a prime example of how copycats invent a difference between themselves and Atkins. The South Beach Diet has been marketed as a "healthier" Atkins, while conjuring fashionable images of tropical beaches and bikini-clad bodies. However, actual comparisons of menus published in *Atkins for Life* and *The South Beach Diet* reveal few differences. Indeed, independent analysis of the meal plans shows no statistical difference between Atkins and South Beach in levels of healthy fats and nutrient-rich carbs. And yes, that includes the amount of saturated fat included in a typical week's menu for both programs. The suggestion that the South Beach program offers a lower-fat or healthier-fat approach is simply inaccurate.

> *The bottom line is that the public needs a healthy approach to eating based on peer-reviewed science, not variations named after stylish beaches, or wherever. Individuals and groups seeking to cash in on the growing interest in controlled-carb nutrition will probably always cook up "new" weight-loss programs hyped by catchy terminology and be set apart by negligible changes that are touted as "groundbreaking."*

Unfortunately, the confusion and disappointing results consumers may experience because of these false variations could cause them to abandon low-carb nutrition altogether. We cannot let propaganda and what simply sounds good replace science. A proper low-carbohydrate nutritional approach is not about subtle differences in fat grams or exotic oils; *it is about controlling carbohydrates.* And when it comes to that, Atkins is the only time-tested and scientifically validated program in existence.

*As with any new diet and fitness plan, be sure to check with your physician before you begin.

Chapter 11

The Diet That's Right for You

"The difference between the right word and a similar word is the difference between lightning and a lightning bug."

—Mark Twain, American author and humorist

The difference between following a diet that will help you lose weight once and for all—and following the same old, same old fruitless diet dogma that's been around for ages and hasn't ever really worked for you or anyone else like you—is the difference between finally getting healthy or staying fatly, embarrassingly the same. There is science behind the right diet, as shown in the previous chapters.

People always ask me what I eat in a day's time, specifically for each meal, that helps me keep my 150 pounds off.

"It's always different," I answer. "Gimme a for instance."

"Well, like, what did you eat this morning for breakfast - and then lunch?" they might probe.

I always have a little morning pre-walk/pre-workout snack, never a full-blown breakfast; bagels, cereal, or oatmeal anymore. And it varies according to what I'm in the mood for or what's on hand. Some days it's three pieces of hard salami and a few almonds. Other days it could be a couple of razor-slim slices of Prosciutto di Parma with a fat, finger-sized slab of Italian Friulano cheese, low-fat cheddar or string cheese, all with a palm-full of almonds, pistachios or cashews.

Usually in mid-afternoon I have a wonderfully crunchy, low-glycemic apple and a few more nuts for bread-crust-like texture, mouth feel and crunch. Almonds, pistachios, and cashews are lifesavers in more ways than one. Sinfully delicious, wonderful for keeping your cholesterol in check, pop a few in your mouth with almost any food to trick your mind into thinking you're actually eating a crusty piece of Italian bread. Helped me kick the bread habit.

I've been known to go through a two-pound bag of almonds or a 16-ounce jar of cashews about every two weeks. When you come visit me, you will find that I always keep a cute cupful of each of these three nut varieties right on the kitchen counter next to the sink for snacks, as well as a small Ziploc bag of them in my purse, just in case.

After my morning workout and cardio walk, I'm hungry for something filling that will hold me and keep me from grazing till dinner. I might have some tuna and egg salad, salmon salad, or deli meats with nuts, grape tomatoes, and cheese.

I always make sure to eat foods high in protein and try to stay away from the white starchy, sugary carbs as much as I can. *Try* is the operative word here, kids. Like Yoda once told Luke Skywalker: "There is no 'try'—only 'do.'" Now I'm telling you: there is no *try*—only *do*.

The less white starch and sugar you eat, the less you'll wanna eat and the less hungry you'll be. Trust Dr. Atkins, Dr. Agatston of the South Beach Diet fame, and me on this and try it for yourself.

The first thing I look for when choosing anything to eat is the carb content and glycemic index, then I subtract the fiber to get the "net carb" count. I'm more concerned with white starch and sugar carbs, glycemic index, and portion control than anything else.

Make It Easy and Healthy

When I'm on the go, what interests me most diet-wise is a yummy, low-carb meal that is portion controlled, ready to eat in a few microwaved minutes, highly portable, and because it's low-carb, curbs my appetite into the wee hours of the afternoon. If you can tolerate the sodium, low-carb frozen entrees could be an invaluable aid for your weight-loss program. I owe a 150-pound debt of gratitude (in part) to frozen entrees. They certainly weren't all I ate, but they were a successful diet staple that taught me portion control, too.

And please allow me a shameless plug here for Atkins' delicious new low-carb frozen entrees. They're the very best in the marketplace and I would know. They're also the best tasting, have the lowest carb count, and are lowest in sodium, too. As soon as I'm down to my last one, I liberally stock up on them so I won't run out and be tempted to eat something on the spur of the moment that I shouldn't. The Crustless Chicken Pot Pie is killer and I could eat that stuff night after night after night. Just depends how busy I am and how much time I have to actually make something else to eat. But with these delicious, low-carb frozen entrees, why bother to cook at all?

When I first started to lose weight, I'd grab a huge handful of frozen petite French green beans and nuke 'em with the entrée to bulk up the quantity, add fiber, and make myself think I was eating more than I actually was. Which, in fact, I really was.

Now, my stomach's shrunk enough to where I can barely finish a whole frozen entrée with almonds or cashews sprinkled on top. On the days when I'm seriously starving, I go back to the green bean thing. Works like a charm and keeps my face out of a lot of other carb-y crap I shouldn't be eating.

And while you're at it, eat a little slower and learn to savor the flavor.

After all, the difference between the right diet and the same old, same old diet is the difference between lightning and a lightning bug.

Pick the best diet to change your life—for life. If you have no idea about the best diet for you, your doctor should offer some advice about a healthy, effective eating plan and what kind of daily exercise you are able to endure to help you get on with your new, healthier lifestyle—for life. Once you get your medical issues under control, and your doc's okay, I can help you with your diet, your motivation and the rest.

Part Three

Create Your Own Weight-Loss Story

Chapter 12

Powerful Questions to Get You Thinking About Saving Your Life

"The only way of finding the limits of the possible is by going beyond them into the impossible."

—*Arthur C. Clarke, British science fiction author, inventor, and futurist*

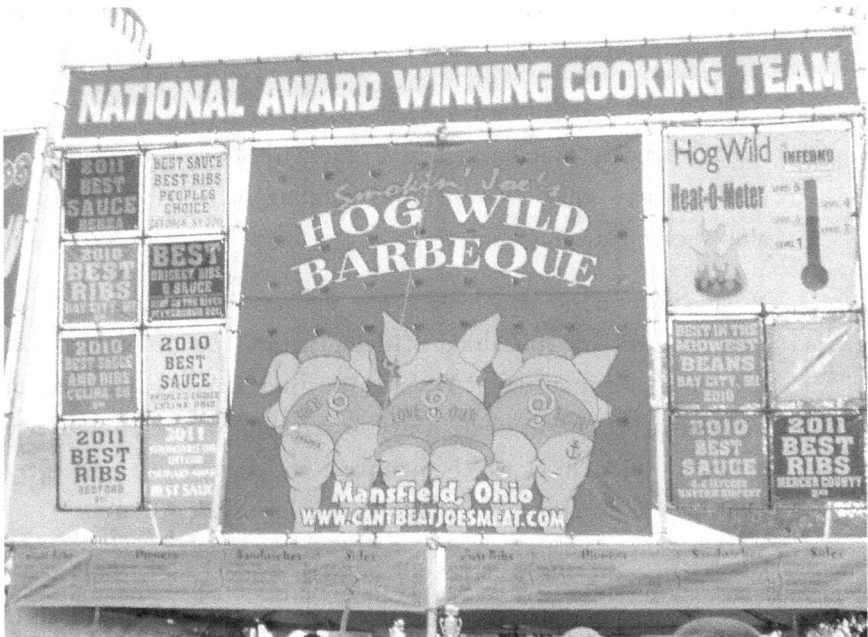

What are you eating that's keeping you fat? Because, no matter what you think to the contrary, you wear what you eat. Look in the mirror. What do you see? Think about what you are doing (or not doing) that's keeping you fat. Because it surely is something; possibly too many white, starchy, sugary carbs and not moving enough every day. Tell me I'm wrong …

Now take the time to answer the following questions that are designed to help you help yourself.

1. What is really important to you in your life?

2. Where do you want to be by the end of the year with your weight, health, and fitness?

3. What needs to be different in order for you to become more healthy and fit?

4. How can I help you find the secret to your own true and everlasting weight loss once and for all? Because it is possible.

5. When will you be ready to "Commit To Get Fit"? When will you be ready to give up all your excuses and just begin your new diet and fitness plan, before it's too late?

6. What's holding you back? Think about this one long and hard because there surely is something standing in your way—and in almost every case, it's y-o-u.

7. What concerns do you have about the possible consequences of your weight? Are you afraid of dying before you get to see your grandkids and spoil them? Perhaps your mom and/or dad died far too young because of being heavy or refusing to give up whatever unhealthy lifestyle in which they were entrenched that cost them their lives. How closely are you following in their footsteps?

8. What concerns do you have regarding your health and being overweight, other than the usual things such as high blood pressure, Type 2 diabetes, heart disease, cancer, or stroke?

9. What concerns do you have regarding your close personal relationships? Do you fear that if you lost weight your spouse,

COMMIT TO GET FIT

significant other, or whomever won't like you, won't love you anymore? What if they will like you and love you even more once you get healthy and more fit, so you could share more fully in all the life activities that make up your relationship? No more sitting it out on the sidelines.

10. What are you afraid of? What scares you the most about losing weight and becoming the person you've always longed to be? Why are you letting the fear of losing weight and becoming more fit stand in your way?

11. How are you going to make the most of yourself and your diet, health, and fitness resources going forward?

12. What does your life look like with regard to your diet, health, and daily cardio in the near future? What does your life look like in the next six months? In the next year? In five years, if you're lucky enough to live that long, hauling all that weight around?

13. What will it take for your inner sparks of possibility to be fanned into the flames of desire and achievement for better health, daily walking, and a new, happier, healthier, slimmer, more fit you—for life?

14. What diet are you willing to go on right now? If you still haven't decided on a healthy, effective diet,* then choose the one that has previously worked the best for you in the past. It's time to seriously consider going on that diet ASAP. Or, finish reading this book and follow the recommendations. You can also think about hiring me as your personal motivational weight-loss coach so that we can work together to help you do exactly what I have done for myself and hundreds of others just like us: find the secret to your own true and everlasting weight loss, once and for all.

Here are a few things to consider: You must be able to stay on your new diet/eating plan from Monday through Friday once you lose all your unhealthy, unwanted weight, in order to keep it off forever. Just know that if you go back to your old eating habits and couch-potato ways by not walking every day, your weight will creep right back on—by the handfuls. You know it. I know it. You've probably lived it for a whole lifetime, just like I did. I'm living proof of what is possible.

And I will say this much: You have to exercise daily* for as long as you're able to move, because there isn't any other way for you to get your weight off and keep it off forever. Dieting alone will not do the trick. And surely you've discovered by now that you cannot exercise away a bad diet.

And please don't even try to use the excuse that you're too stressed and don't have time to think about losing weight, getting fit, or doing any other healthy stuff right now. We're all under a tremendous amount of pressure and stress these days; you're not alone. Using stress and other external matters as excuses to evade the issue is counterproductive. And excuses turn into denials.

All I can tell you is the only way to find the limits of what's possible with regard to your weight loss and wellness is by going beyond them into the impossible. Make up your mind to be honest with yourself from now on and begin again right now, right where you are. While there's still time.

*As with any new diet and fitness plan, be sure to check with your physician before you begin.

Chapter 13

Acquire the Desire

"Obstacles can't stop you. Problems can't stop you. Most of all, other people can't stop you. Only you can stop you."

—*Jeffrey Gitomer, American author and sales trainer*

Years ago, a good friend of mine was in big trouble—she couldn't seem to stop eating. Every time I saw her, which wasn't very often because she lived in another city, she appeared to be packing on more pounds.

My rapidly expanding friend then visited another good gal pal of ours who called me in pure panic with the report. She begged me to send our girlfriend one of my motivational, come-to-Jesus, kick-in-the-butt, lose-weight-now-or-die-before-your-time e-mails that I'm known to send from time to time to keep many of you and a lot of my friends motivated, reminding all y'all to eat right, walk, or do some other form of cardio an hour a day to lose weight and get healthier. This is all it takes to shed those ugly, unhealthy, unwanted pounds you've been hauling around with you since, maybe, forever.

My friend needs to get a serious grip and only she can do it. I can prod all I want, but she needs to be sick of schlepping herself around. She needs to be sick of squeezing into way too-tight pants, skirts, and tops. She needs to be sick of her husband's humiliating, disparaging remarks. She needs to be sick of the way she looks—like an old bag before her time—and the way she feels—probably like an even older bag.

She also needs to acknowledge that she's addicted to white starch and sugar and that's probably why her eating is so totally out of control. She has to break her insidious carb addiction. A modified, low-fat Atkins Diet did it for me and continues to keep my weight from piling back on.

My friend needs to take the horse by its hair and do something about her self-destructive eating behavior. I've been there a time or two, myself, so I know what she's going through. She has to stop hurting herself with food and drink. Neither she nor her husband would dare miss an evening cocktail hour, but daily cardio? Fugeddaboudit. "No time," is her/his/their excuse.

She has to learn to close her mouth and mind to all that useless junk, the white, starchy, sugary carbs she's stuffing and poisoning her body with. It's those crafty carbs that fool us into thinking they comfort us, when they really keep us addicted and crawling helplessly back for more.

In the meantime, she, and maybe you, too, need to hop on that scale, burn those numbers you see between your chubby little feet right into your brain, take a long, hard look at yourself in the mirror—right smack in the eye, actually—and promise yourself to take immediate steps to do something about your health, weight, fitness, and appearance. Prontito.

If you're anything like my friend, you need to begin walking—and I mean serious daily walking—even if it's just around the health club, horse farm, beach, or block at first. Even if it's only twenty minutes a day for the first week or two; it's all a matter of developing the daily habit. You gotta start somewhere. And you gotta do it every day for thirty-five straight days to develop the habit.

No excuses. Nothing and no one is worth damaging yourself through overeating. Begin to love yourself more than anyone or anything else on this still-green Earth: more than your husband, significant other, kids, or carbs themselves. In the long run, you are all you have and all that matters.

Regardless of where you are with your weight, fitness and eating, you can begin to turn things around right now. But you really gotta wanna ... What's the absolute worst that could happen to you if you lost weight? You'd be healthier. You'd move more easily, compared to how you feel right now when you move, or walk, or go to the bathroom, or climb a flight of stairs, or get in and out of a car, or whatever.

And those aches and pains you have? Gone, or nearly so, once you get all that junk outta your trunk. Keep your chin up, your eyes straight ahead, and take the whole thing meal by meal, step by step, pound by precious pound. There is no other way.

You have to acquire the desire to change, to get better, healthier, slimmer, more fit, more active, more attractive, more vital, more lively, more spry, more agile, more vibrant, more beautiful, more of everything. Get the picture?

Make One Better Choice Every Day

Recently, while cardio-rowing at the club, I was lamenting to Margaret Posh, one of my Goddess-Girlfriends, about how I'd love to knock off a few more pounds then call it a day and maintain that weight for life when up walks one of Margaret's own Goddess-Girlfriends, a gal named Kathy, who looks exactly like Gabrielle Reece, the gorgeously tall, statuesque, Olympic volleyball champ who's married to Laird Hamilton, the equally gorgeous, internationally renowned, extreme surfing champion.

Gabrielle, I mean, Kathy, then plunks down on the rowing machine just to my right, Margaret was on my left and I found myself squeezed between these two gals, sort of like a Goddess sandwich with me as the minced meat in the middle.

Anyway, while we rowed, we got to talking chocolate and both gals fessed up, much to my surprise, that they eat chocolate every single day - OMG! - and still manage to look the way they do.

I mean, you wouldn't expect ladies who look like these two to indulge in a daily dependence on chocolate. Looking at each of them, who would ever think they let the stuff pass through their luscious lips, but they do.

"How do you control it, the addiction?" I asked. "You know, so it doesn't get the better of you and pack on unwanted pounds?"

Each looked at the other and laughed. "We're very, very selective with what we eat and all our other food choices are healthy, and organic when possible. And we keep an eye on everything else we eat. We eat to live, we don't live to eat. Food is fuel. And we workout every single day, just like you do!" they said, almost in unison.

"Well then, why don't I look like you two?" I laughed.

Margaret reminded me to get back to making at least one better, healthier choice every day. And when I'm reaching for a piece of Dove milk chocolate, rethink the choice and make a better selection. Do it once, just for one day. Then the next day, do it again, and again the day after that, reminding yourself to make better, healthier choices every day.

Well, you know me, one day turned into the next and I made better choices the second day, too. And after a week, I ran into Margaret at the club and when I told her how I got through the last seven days, she smiled and asked how I felt.

"Confident," I replied, "and in control, which is what it took for me to shed 150 pounds of unwanted weight in the first place. I developed control. I'm still in control. And I also do an hour of daily cardio without fail, which is another control issue. And it makes me feel fabulous, because I'm in control."

When you control exactly what you eat and how much you move every day, nothing can stand in your way. You run the show. You call the shots with regard to your own weight, health, and fitness—and eventually everything else, really. You gain confidence when you're in total control and then the sky's the limit.

Now, you can do what you have to do and sometimes you can do it even better than you think you can. Make just one better, healthier choice in your eating and fitness routines today. Prove to yourself that you can do it. Learn to be in even better control of yourself than you think you can.

Set Three Clear and Measurable Weight-Loss Goals

In order to succeed in any weight-loss and wellness plan, you have to set clear weight-loss and wellness goals *and* reinforce them each and every day. What do you want to achieve? Maybe you want to walk or run a faster lap? Got a yen for a quicker step? Wanna lose twenty, forty, 100 pounds, or more? How about being able to walk for an hour straight without gasping or needing a nap afterward?

These things could very well happen for you, but your first step is to define your three most important weight-loss and wellness goals by writing them down and/or stating them out loud to your friends, family, coworkers, boss, class, or me, your new motivational weight-loss coach. Tell someone who will remember your intentions, remind you about them, and hold you accountable—daily, if need be.

When you "go public" with your goals, it's hard to break the contract you set up with yourself and others. It gets really embarrassing when you don't stick to your goal. Makes you appear weak. Undisciplined. Unmotivated to improve your health and fitness no matter what your mouth says.

The difference between a goal and a daydream is that the goal requires action to achieve. The daydream happens the rest of the time, while we're sitting on the sofa, driving, or just contemplating what to eat next.

1. *Write your weight loss and wellness goals in your fitness journal and also post them where you'll see them the most: fridge, freezer, bathroom mirror, or your computer screen. Sticky note them to your dashboard or your forehead - places like that. Keep those goals right in your face day after day.*

2. The next step is to *give yourself a reasonable deadline.* You can use my trick with important events, holidays, and other significant events: I count backward from the deadline or date and set daily points of reference on my calendar to keep myself on track along the way. The countdown really helps. Creating smaller, incremental goals to motivate yourself as you go will help keep you on your path to both weight loss and improved health. Don't go for the whole enchilada right off the bat.

When you write them down, your goals become your reason and your road map—the *why* you're doing it in the first place. Make everything you do count toward your end game, your objective of improved health, fitness, weight loss, and wellness. *Commit to Get Fit* can help you figure out *how* that fits in with your daily lifestyle but only you know the *why,* and only you can do the diet and daily cardio.

Walk, weigh yourself, and record it every single day. Use everything you have at your fingertips as motivation. Nothing else matters if we don't have better health and fitness. How can we help others, how can we help our families and friends, if we can't help ourselves?

Develop Your Own Fitness-Training Routine*

Will Rogers said, "Even if you are on the right track, you'll get run over if you just sit there." Whether it's walking, running, swimming, or working in the gym, begin to develop a daily fitness/cardio routine for yourself right down to what you're going to wear to beat the heat. If you are doing your cardio outside, slather sunscreen on your face, neck, and arms, but do keep it away from your forehead. Wear a hat instead, because that stuff stings worse than the Dead Sea's saltwater when you sweat and it leaks into your eyes.

It is recommended to push yourself to go further and faster with your cardio on at least one day over the weekend. The idea is to stretch your capabilities so your physical performance the following week will benefit.

You'll notice your walks will be a tad easier, you'll do them in a bit faster time and be smiling and feeling strong at the end of each daily jaunt.

All this isn't a gift of genius, or rocket science; it's just common sense.

*As with any new diet and fitness plan, be sure to check with your physician before you begin.

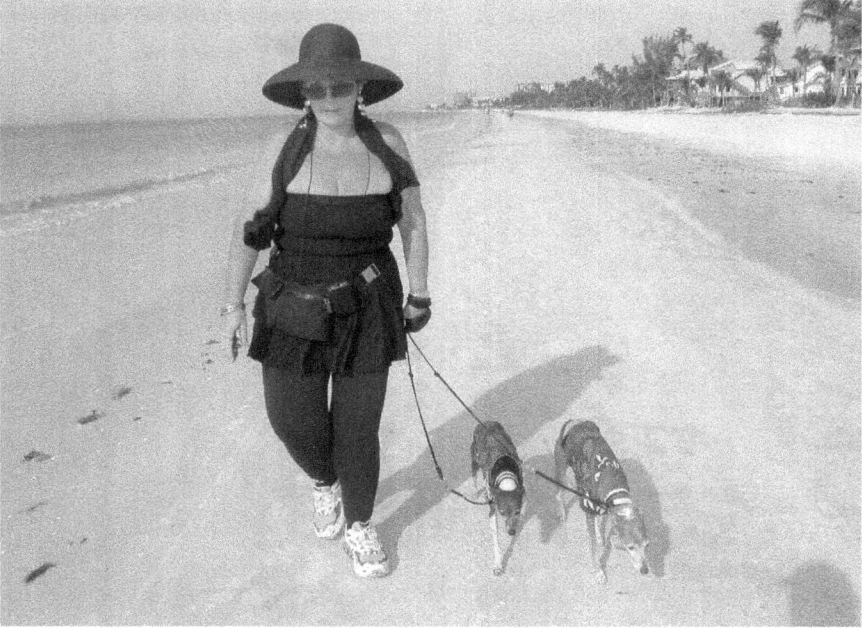

Chapter 14

If a 2,000-Pound Cow Can Take a Walk, You Can, Too

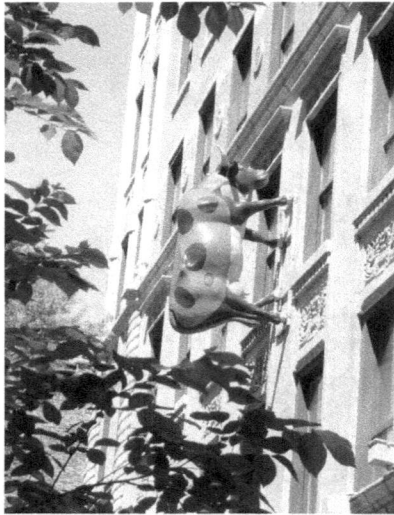

"Until you get dissatisfied, you won't do anything to really move your life to another level. Dissatisfaction is a gem. If you're totally satisfied, you're going to get comfortable. And then your life begins to deteriorate."

—Anthony Robbins, American life coach, self-help author and
motivational speaker

Sometimes I wonder what drives me, what keeps me pounding that pavement day after day after day. Then I look in the mirror and see what daily walking does for me. Then I get on the scale. Then I get it.

Why should *you* take up daily walking? Because it reduces all of the obvious medical risk factors for heart disease, diabetes, and certain cancers.*

Because you'll be able to get around better.

Because you'll finally be able to join your family and friends in lots of other activities instead of sitting it out on the sidelines because it's too difficult for you to move the way you are now.

Because you can't swim to the grocery store.

Because it can be done anywhere, at any time.

Because you can walk whenever and wherever you want.

Because you'll see something fun, new, and amazing every day.

Because you can walk alone, with your dog, accompanied by a friend, in a group, or on your way to and from work.

Because you can walk on your lunch hour.

Because you don't need special equipment, just the best pair of walking shoes you can afford.

Because walking leaves you exhilarated.

Because it makes you stronger physically - as well as mentally and emotionally.

Because you can always tell the diligent daily walkers from the sometime strollers because they have on serious walking shoes and bigger smiles than anyone else.

Because the more you walk, the less you'll want to overeat. I still can't believe it, and I'm in my tenth consecutive year of daily fitness walking, but it is true.

Because instead of eating as the one thing you do the best when all else fails, you can now control it through your daily walking. Take a walk instead of stuffing yourself.

Because it's way more satisfying to your psyche and less damaging to your body than overeating - not to mention the incredible health, fitness, and appearance benefits you'll gain. But I already said that, didn't I?

Because you will finally be able to show your husband, wife, lover, pal, significant other, partner, kids, mom, stepdad, and *yourself* who's boss.

Take that daily walk because, like everything else in life, it's all up to you. Walk daily for the health of it. Walk daily for your life. You can't direct the wind, that's for sure. But you certainly can readjust your sails until you find the right combination of diet and daily cardio that's the perfect fit for you.*

Walk for Your Life

I began walking daily in earnest January 1, 2003. They say it takes thirty-five straight days to make or break a habit. At the time, we were in Florida for several weeks, so I had the luxury of the wonderful warmer weather to help me.

I also had to enlist the aid of my husband and two mini Italian Greyhound rescues, "Mama needs your help, kids. She can't do this alone. It's far too painful, so you have to come with me," I implored.

About the tenth or eleventh day into my new daily cardio walking regimen, it was raining like it was the end of the world. Literally. This was no tropical drizzle, trust me. It was a full-blown, on-the-verge-of-being-a-monsoon rain. As I raced through the house with my umbrella, desperate to get out the door before I chickened out, my husband said to me, "Where are you going?"

"Walking," I replied.

"It's pouring!" he protested.

"Look, today's my tenth consecutive day of walking. I've never managed to do ten consecutive days of anything in my whole life let alone cardio walking. If I don't do my hour's walk today and it's raining tomorrow, and if I choose not to walk tomorrow, that'll be two days missed, and then if it's still raining the third day from now and I don't take that walk—I'll be finished before I even really got started. So I *have* to walk every single day, regardless of the weather."

He told me to hold on, that he was getting his umbrella and coming with me. When we returned to Chicago from Florida that February, I panicked when I realized I had walked about forty days straight without missing a step in the Florida winter's heat—and now I was confronted with Chicago's famous frigid temps. I said to myself, *You used to ski when it was 30° below zero, so if you could get out and ski in that, you can certainly get your butt out the door to take your hour's cardio walk every day regardless of the climatic conditions.*

Next thing I knew, I dug out my old ski clothes, goggles and mitts, slipped into my Under Armor cold gear tights, and took my first walk in Chicago's Windy City winter's wind.

In all fairness to walking in inclement weather, I've had some of the most incredibly beautiful, meditative, invigorating walks in the crappiest of conditions. Something about softly lit, low-lying clouds, fog, and snow drizzle stimulates the senses. You will learn to cherish these daily walks and use them to meditate and discover things about yourself and your surroundings you never saw before.

And that's exactly how I started my daily cardio walking practice.* If you can't make yourself take that walk every day, I don't know what to tell you. It's the least you can do to take care of yourself, and you're missing out on so much more than just the cardio bennies.

Woody Allen is said to walk eight miles a day. Why? Certainly not to keep his already svelte frame but to benefit from all that subconscious stimulation so that when he goes back to his desk, he's more centered and productive creatively.

It can be the same for you, too. Got something ailing you, really under your skin, bothering you? Wanna smack your boss, spouse, or kid to kingdom come? Take that cardio walk today not only for the health of it, but to ease your spirit, mind and soul. You will thank yourself for it.

Since I began walking in earnest, I've managed to walk over 35,000 miles, or one and one-third times around the Earth at the equator, leaving about 150 pounds in my wake. I urge you to do the same.

And if you can't sustain a daily cardio practice, ask yourself why? Are you really just too dang lazy? Are you waiting for someone else to do it for you? News Flash: ain't gonna happen. Just like you cannot exercise away a bad diet, no one can get out there and do your daily cardio for you, either. By measuring what you do cardio- and weight-wise on a daily basis, you will discover any weaknesses or inconsistency in your routine and nip that laziness right in the bud. If you wanna.

Or else you're doomed to stay overweight and unhealthy forever, because if you're severely overweight, you are unhealthy. No question about it. There is no such thing as a healthy 300-plus pound person who is 5'2" tall. Sorry.

Start by becoming aware of your exercise-less behavior and pay attention. Many more surprising opportunities to squeeze your daily cardio in here and there will present themselves to you if you just open up your mind and eyes. It's up to you not to ignore these opportunities and get the message.

By becoming aware of what you're doing with your time, the excuses you're making for NOT taking that fifteen to twenty minute lunchtime walk that will allow you to squeeze in one-third of your daily cardio will become crystal clear to you.

Look at my before and after pictures to see what I looked like when I first started walking, and I wasn't even my fattest in that picture. Then see what I looked like a year later and what I look like now, down about 150 pounds since I started. Nothing like a visual to snap you back to reality.

Turn THIS

Into THIS

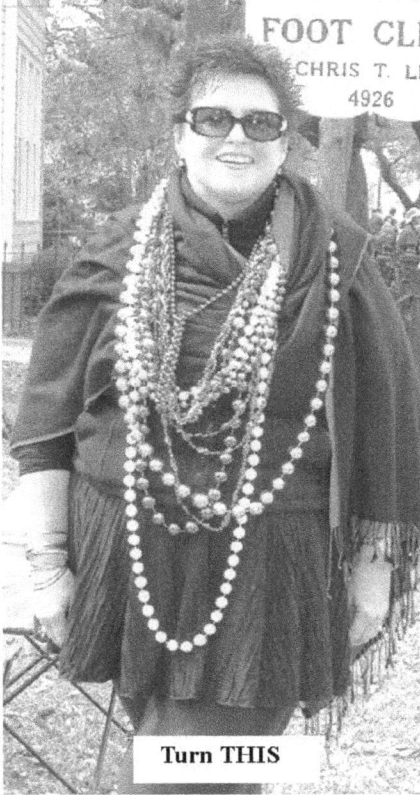

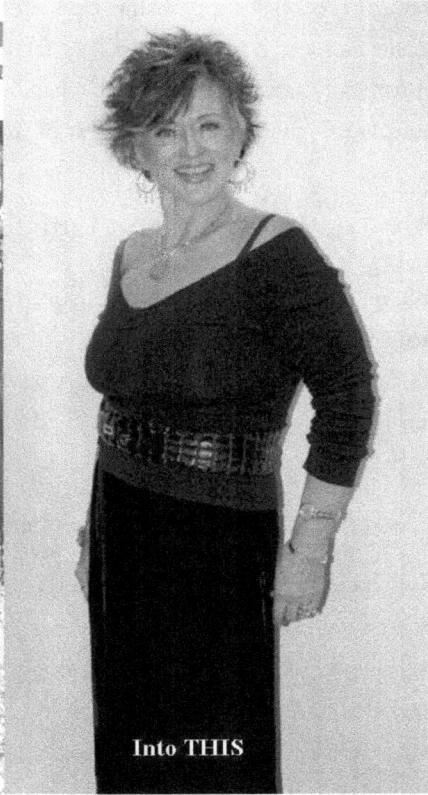

Lately, I've seen too many people fail in their attempts to lose their weight once and for all through last-ditch efforts of gastric bypass, strict liquids only, and a lot of other fad diets in which the participants are assured lasting results without daily exercise. Phooey. It ain't so. Just ask anyone who's managed to get it off and keep it off for this long.

I'll walk outside and in almost any type of weather conditions to get my daily walk in because I don't ever want to go back to being fat again.

Weighing myself *every* day helps me to never let my weight escalate up past four or five pounds, Period. And that's happened only once since I began. I wasn't vigilant in my daily weighing, and before I knew it, my weight was up about ten pounds.

You just know I nipped that right in the bud as soon as I saw it and vowed to never let it happen again. It's far too easy and dangerous for a formerly chronically obese person to backslide. I am determined to keep a healthy handle on my weight for the rest of my life.

Are You In or Are You Out?

We're all in this together. The number one question I'm always asked is how I finally got motivated to successfully lose 130 pounds in two and a half years, and how I continue to stay motivated to keep it off now into my tenth year, even managing to shed about another twenty pounds between both knee replacement rehabs.

"You really gotta wanna," is always my reply.

You have to be sick and tired of hauling yourself around, of being out of breath, of not being able to take a long walk with less pain than you feel right now, of not being able to easily get up from a chair. You just have to hate the state you're in and be ready to do whatever it takes, and I do mean whatever it takes once and for all, to lose your excess weight and be healthier and more fit. You have to become laser-focused and unstoppable. No matter what.

Different things motivate different people. You have to find out what motivates you. For me, it was the fact that I'd finally had enough. It was time for drastic action. My main motive, however, was being sick of the way I looked and felt. At 317 pounds and rapidly climbing, I was literally tired of hauling myself around. It was just too much damn work. And for what?

There may be times over the coming months when it might become difficult to lose your weight, but hang in there. It does begin to move again, sooner or later depends on how diligent you are with monitoring your daily carb intake and cardio walking. The more determined you are with your efforts, the faster they'll pay off.

Life is only as tough as we want to make it. As the saying goes: "Pick your own kind of hard." The same can be said for making a serious lifestyle change. It's not as difficult as you might think once you get started, but getting started is no cakewalk, either. It does take determination, effort, and daily vigilance, and you've got to get out of your denial about how unfit and unhealthy you really are.

I can tell you from experience that it's well worth the effort. Whatever sacrifice you have to make, whatever fave foods you have to give up, it's all well worth it in the end. And remember: I need to constantly motivate myself to sail successfully through my days, too. I take it one step at a time. One meal at a time. One cardio session at a time. One pound at a time. One day at a time.

And don't even try to tell me you're comfortable just the way you are. Are you kidding? You wouldn't be reading this book if you felt comfortable and loved yourself the way you should.

Stop your denial.

Stop your unhappiness and dissatisfaction.

Stop your deterioration because that's exactly what being overweight is: gross, negligent deterioration.

It's all up to you to move your life to another, healthier level. It's your personal responsibility.

Let's get started. Are you in or are you out?

*As with any new diet and fitness plan, be sure to check with your physician before you begin.

Chapter 15

Cardio Boxing's a Blast, or How Three Inglorious Little Basterds Taught a Boomer Babe the Finer Points of Life in the Cardio Fast Lane

"The first step in getting what you want out of life is this: Decide what you want."

—Ben Stein, American actor, writer, lawyer, and commentator on political and economic issues

More and more people ask me what else they can do to help reinvigorate their diet and fitness plans throughout the year, but with a new spin on it because they're getting a bit bored with their usual routine. "Like, what else would *you* personally do for daily cardio?" they want to know.

Well, with the help of a few guy pals from East Bank Club, I found an exciting alternative to the customary cardio choices out there and one recent Monday, my own cardio routine took an unexpected hit: I had my first "official," professional boxing lesson with Glen Freedman, the club's boxing coach extraordinaire and two of his astute and cute students, Howard and Pat (a guy).

Let me just say this much: when I decided to send them an e-mail of thanks for the experience later that evening, I could barely move. By 6:45 p.m., my shoulders screamed in their sockets, and by 8:00 p.m., I could barely lift my arms and eyelids at all.

As the temporary (I hoped) paralysis slowly progressed down the rest of my body and I realized I couldn't move a muscle, let alone think to type an e-mail, I unintentionally crashed until the next morning.

Boxing's definitely cardio in the fast lane and not for the faint of heart, nor weak-muscled—make no mistake about that. But if you're looking for an intense cardio burn to revive or jump-start your daily workouts, and you think you can handle it physically, boxing could be just the ticket.

Let me just say that I barely got through the rest of my weight workout after our lesson ended, staggering around the club trying to get my bearings and keeping my eyeballs from spinning smack out of my head. It was that intense of a workout experience for me.

And don't get me wrong, after sweating like a guy with the guys for an hour, I totally blew off my usual daily hour's cardio cross-train on the rowing machine and treadmill. I figured enough cardio is enough for one day. I warmed up, pre-boxing, so I knew I was in really good shape, cardio-wise, for the day. I just wasn't in really good shape otherwise.

I'm sure I'd get used to the impact on my shoulder and upper back bones eventually, but the rope jumping also has me beat for now. I can't seem to spring myself into the air like I used to, but I'm sure I'll get the hang of it with some practice should I choose to continue.

However, when I told my Russian physical therapist/personal trainer/naprapath, Sergey, that I flunked the jump rope portion of my lesson, he said in his inimitable Russian accent, "Vy vould you vant to do zat, anyvay? I ztrongly vould recommend you didn't even try zat vit your hiztory!"

Looks like if I want to continue, I might have to find an alternative to the boxer's traditional rope jumping warm-ups and between-set practice. But what Sergey really meant vas, I mean was: Vy vould I even vant to jeopardize my physical abilities such as they are, to take on boxing?

In my heart I knew he was right. Sergey's originally from the Soviet Union and used to train a lot of their Olympic athletes back in the day, before all this state-of-the-art fitness equipment we have available now.

So you can well imagine what Sergey's seen and how well he trains me and all the rest of his clients. And you can also imagine what a wealth of health and wellness information he is, too. That said, he knows my physical limitations almost better than I do because he's a doctor of naprapathy and has been with me through several of my knee surgeries, countless physical therapy rehabs, and all. And we both know that besides keeping my daily walking stamina up, I need to do a lot of non-weight-bearing cardio as often as possible.

So meanwhile, back at my first and last boxing lesson: the best part of the session next to the sweating, punching and the boy ballet of ducking and dodging was listening to the guys "man-versations," one of my all-time personal fave pastimes who stems from growing up surrounded by nothing but boys, I'm sure.

Of course, I'm dramatizing this a bit, but boxing is a form of cardio in a much bigger way than what I'm used to or almost anything else that I've ever done. It ranks right up there with rock wall climbing and the triathlon as far as the sweat and exertion factors are concerned, and uses every single muscle in your entire body like these other activities do, as well.

Boxing's allure was an out-of-the-norm, more intense cardio burn, and I sure got more than I bargained for.

What was it that my mother used to tell me? Something about curiosity killing the cat?

As I mentioned, I found I used muscles I haven't used in decades, perspired like I haven't since I helped build the Pyramids, and can see where this boxing thing is a really terrific workout for those physically capable of handling the impact on their body. But, sadly, I am not.

And, wow, those guys sure do work up a super sweat of their own. Howard had rivers of it running off his nose. And our fellow boxer, Pat, on the other hand, moved like a butterfly and stung like Ali.

A tip: if you're a mildly OCD germ freak, you might want to purchase your own wrist and hand wraps as the tapes used on me were a tad "gym-y smelling," if you know what I mean.

The musky scent I whiffed throughout the lesson harkened me back to the days of walking into Chicago Vocational High School's gym during wrestling practice. And, well, let me just say, I couldn't beat a path to the Ladies Room fast enough after class to wash up to my armpits with soap. But that's just me.

Once Glen wrapped my delicately sensitive artist's hands with great care, he gingerly slid red, 16-ounce boxing gloves on me for extra protective padding. So, in addition to swinging, punching, and pumping my arms in ways I'm not normally used to, I had one-pound "weights" Velcro-ed to each of my own lovely little mitts.

Then there was the "jewelry thing" for me to contend with. Those who know me, know it took a few minutes for me to de-bracelet and de-ring myself. Why I don't think ahead in these circumstances is beyond me. With my regular walking and cardio routines, I don't have to remove a thing. I don't even have to think. For wall/rock climbing and boxing, all the swinging, jangly jewels and accessories have to go. One could lose a dainty digit or an errant earlobe if not careful.

At the end of the hour, just when you think the clock has almost run out and you're home free, Glen pulls yet another pro trainer's trick out of his boxing bag and makes each student lie on the floor, on their back, and do abs and core work that would dust the average individual, had I not had the privilege of six straight years of once a week, private Pilates lessons under my belt.

Heh-heh, I thought, as Glen and the other two boys stared at me open-mouthed. Pilates gives you a super-strong core when done right and I love what it's done for me as a non-impact modality: improved my physical fitness and balance, and increased my strength.

When you come right down to it, a lot in life is all about having a strong core, and that's no bull. And, man, what a lesson I got that day, not only in boxing, but in life skills, as well.

So, as I said, by 6:45 p.m., all I wanted to do was kill those Three Inglorious Little Boxing Basterds. Every single muscle, every fiber, every follicle, and nanometer of my body hurt. Not only from the vigorous punching and jabbing, but from using parts of my frame that have been asleep for a long, long while. All right, I hurt from the laughing, too.

From what I've heard and observed, I have a new respect for all three boys. This Boomer Babe discovered that boxing is a Zen-like experience of life in the cardio fast lane - all while getting one's butt kicked, metaphorically speaking, of course.

Chapter 16

Swimming

"You can do what you have to do, and sometimes you can do it even better than you think you can."

—*Jimmy Carter, 39th President of the United States*

You can't find a better overall type of exercise for your cardiovascular fitness than in water activities like swimming and water aerobics. It's low impact on your joints, it burns the greatest amount of calories compared to land-based exercise, and it's fun. Who doesn't like swimming and being in a pool?

Let's go over some facts about water and why exercising in water takes more energy. Water is substantially denser than air, so it has a much greater resistance to motion through it. When you move your arm across your body under water, it encounters approximately fifteen times more resistance than moving it through air. Therefore, your muscles have to work much harder and burn more calories doing so.

Your body will lose considerably more heat through water than through air. The exchange of heat from your body to water is about twenty-five times greater than through air. Your body has to generate more heat and burn more calories if you are in water than if you are on land at the same temperature. If you stand on land when the temperature is 82°, you may feel comfortable or even slightly warm. Being in 82° water up to your neck, you will likely feel cool.

Why Swimming Is Easy on Your Body

The buoyancy of water reduces the impact of stress on your joints by up to 90% more than land-based exercises. The water is pushing up against your body as compared to being on land where only gravity is acting on your body. The buoyancy of water is particularly beneficial for those individuals who have arthritis, joint trauma, or need rehabilitation from an injury. (I rehabbed my butt off in water after every single one of my knee surgeries, trust me on this. Where there's a will, there's a way, and water was it for me for awhile.) The supporting force of water is also great for pregnant women who want to continue to exercise, the elderly, obese people who can't handle the joint stress of walking or running, and very young children, as well.

Water is not as solid as land, so creating motion through it requires a great deal more energy to create forward movement. When you walk or run on land, your foot pushes off against a solid surface and creates a forward motion. In water, it is much harder to create that forward motion. Since water is fluid, it moves in all directions and does not remain steady when a force is applied against it. It moves away from the force. So when you try to swim, your hand catches the water in front of you, pulls it back toward you and you pull your body forward. However, the water is slipping around your hand because it is not firm like grabbing a rope in front of you to pull.

You are expending a lot of energy to create minimal forward movement and you burn more calories to do so. Your body is also expending energy just to overcome the resistance of water as well. You require a greater deal of energy to move the same distance through water than walk or run on land. The world record for the 100-meter men's freestyle is about forty-seven seconds and the world record for running the men's 100-meter dash is about 9.6 seconds. And yet, the swimmer will burn about three times as many calories to cover the same distance.

How to Start Swimming

In the Swimming Appendix at the end of this book, there are links to various swimming organizations, magazines, accessories, and places to swim to help you locate what you need. The most likely places to get started with your in-water exercise program should be close to where you live. Most high schools with swimming pools offer swim aerobics, may have open swim times, or sponsor a local USA Swimming chartered swim club for children and Masters Swimming (adult) swim clubs. You can also find these aqua programs and many more at several other locations in your area, such as the YMCA or YWCA organizations, your park district or community recreation department, most of the national health clubs, country clubs, etc. All have swim related activities to explore.

At any of these places with swimming pools, there should be instructors to help you get started and also teach you the correct stroke, body position, breathing techniques, etc. If you haven't swum in a long time or are new to swimming, please remember that this will take time. Do not get frustrated and do not give up. You have no idea of the poor shape you are in until you get into a swimming pool. You can take the top athletes of all the major sports and put them in a pool and they will struggle to swim 100 meters and likely never get to 500 meters.

No activity takes the energy and endurance requirements like that of swimming. Start slowly and work your way up. Good things come to those who practice with patience. Start with one length of the pool and take a break if you need one. Then do it again over and over until you can't. Rest for a day and do it again. In the beginning, don't try to swim every day because you will be too tired and get frustrated. Start with three days a week. Then the next week, try to do an extra couple lengths. When you are ready, try two continuous lengths of the pool, and then take a short break and try it again. You want to slowly build up your endurance and forget about how long it takes you do it. You can work on speed later after your endurance gets a foothold.

Swim into the Fat-Burning Zone

Since swimming is such a demanding cardiovascular activity, you should monitor your heart rate. Not too fast and not too slow. You want to be in the range of about 70% to 80% of your maximum heart rate. Remember the rule of thumb of subtracting your age from 220 and multiplying that by 70% for your target. If you're just starting out, you can check your own pulse after you finish a lap or wear a heart rate monitor on your wrist and check it. So, let's say you are forty years old; your target heart rate should be $220 - 40 = 180 \times 70\% = 126$ or 144 at the 80% mark.

To get into the fat-burning zone, you first have to burn out the existing carbohydrates stored in your muscle's cells. This requires at least twenty minutes of continuous exercise at those target rates. Again, don't worry about this until your endurance level builds up. Your mission is to increase your endurance, and it may take a month or two or three to do so. So what? You will get there as long as you keep at it and never give up.

Once you are at the point where you can swim for twenty minutes straight, you will start to see some significant results, especially if you are doing this three to five times a week or even every day, if possible. At this stage, you can start to increase your stroke rate to swim faster and consequently burn more calories and lose more weight. If you have ever watched competitive swimming on TV or been to a college swim meet, ask yourself *Have I ever seen an overweight swimmer?* They may have been overweight at one time before they started swimming but they aren't now!

As I said earlier, there are instructors and coaches to help you at these locations but here are some of the basics regarding freestyle swimming that you should concentrate on. To swim efficiently and also to prevent injury caused by continually doing something wrong and developing bad habits, pay attention to the following:

1. Keep your head down (just like they tell you in golf) with your eyes looking down. If you lift your head up, your legs will drop down.

As you breathe to the side, half of your head remains in the water with enough of your head showing to the side for your mouth to clear the water line.

2. You have to exhale with your face in the water because you won't have enough time to exhale and inhale while your face is to the side between strokes. Try to exhale through your nose and the last bit with your mouth just before your mouth comes out of the water to clear the water from around your mouth. Breathe with your stomach and don't try to completely fill your lungs. You won't be able to. Keeping air in your lungs through most of your breathing cycles helps you stay on the surface like an air filled balloon.

3. Keep your centerline straight and don't wiggle like a tadpole when you swim. Your backbone is the framework that your body rotates around and your strength is in your core muscles around your hips.

4. Kick from your hips and not your knees. Knees should not be flexed and keep your feet kind of at ease. If you are not doing the butterfly, backstroke, or breaststroke and just doing the freestyle, don't worry about kicking too much unless you want to sprint. You will get too tired from continuous kicking and in the freestyle, kicking doesn't provide that much forward motion unless you have swim fins on.

5. Elbows lead the hands in the freestyle stroke. Don't let them drop but keep them higher in your reach. Your hands come into play after your elbow can't reach any farther forward. Your hand cuts into the water with fingers pointed forward and slightly down and no space between your fingers. You will pull more water with your fingers next to each other rather than spread apart, so be sure to cup your hands. Cut your hands into the water about shoulder width in front of you.

6. Pull your hand back to your hip and no further and then start your hip roll to begin recovering your hand forward again with your elbow high.

7. The roll of your hips is where your power comes from and permits you to take your breaths. When you roll your hips, try not to dig your shoulder into the water because this will hinder you with your breathing and place your head too low in the water to successfully breathe when you turn your head to the side. It will also slow you down.

If you want to start out easier with just water aerobics or a water-exercise program, then that is your option too. You can start building up some muscle strength and flexibility. Get used to the feel of your body in water by doing this first and then move into actually swimming laps. Most high schools, park districts, health clubs, and country clubs all have some type of water exercise programs. Just call any of these places and ask for the aquatic director or pool manager for information.

Swim Clubs

Swimming is also a fantastic activity to get involved with your children; the earlier children learn to swim, the better. Most towns and cities have local swim clubs that practice out of the local high school, Y, or park district. These clubs are usually under the guidelines and rules of USA Swimming. There are fifty-nine Local Swimming Committees (LSCs) under USA Swimming for all the chartered swim clubs. Most are by state, but California and Texas have multiple LSCs due to the sheer size of those states.

For example, in the state of Illinois, there are over 110 chartered swim clubs as part of USA Swimming and about 15,000 kids under the age of eighteen participate in Illinois. In the U.S., there are approximately 2,800 swim clubs with over 400,000 children as members. There is also Masters Swimming for people over eighteen by various age ranges. There are clubs and meets for Masters Swimming and in the summers there is also Open Water swimming in lakes. These are normally distance swimming meets.

These swim clubs are where our Olympic swimmers learn how to swim correctly as children, compete against others in their age group, and then develop into high school, college, and Olympic swimmers. Links to USA Swimming and other swim organizations are listed in the Swimming Appendix in the back of the book. Your local swim club is a great place for your children to develop goals and learn what competing is about, how to win with dignity and, more importantly, how to lose with dignity. They learn what sportsmanship means and make new friends in the area and in your state. It's a fantastic way to spend time with your kids at weekend meets as a family and share in your children's successes and disappointments. Swimming is a sport that can be participated in all year long. Parents can volunteer to be timers and workers at meets your swim club hosts or take a series of training classes and become a swim meet official.

Along with a sustained exercise program, either in the water or land-based, you have to have a healthy meal plan to go with it. It is extremely difficult to get physically healthy and lose weight, even with daily swimming, if you keep eating a large amount of bad carbohydrates. The perseverance and will power you are now devoting to exercise has to also be maintained with your eating habits as well. You can't do one without the other if you want to realize the results that you are hoping for. If you consistently do both, I guarantee you will be successful with your aquatic weight loss and wellness program. Follow these simple steps and, before you know it, you'll be swimming into the fat burning zone.

My Swimming Inspiration

As a final thought, I'm sure most of you heard or saw on the news the beyond incredible story of Diana Nyad. Diana is a world-famous distance swimmer from Florida. She was the first person in history to swim from

Havana, Cuba, to Key West, Florida, without a protective shark cage. She swam 112 miles through the ocean and battled the gulf-stream current, the wind, and highly poisonous box jellyfish, all without sleeping for fifty-three straight hours. Can any of us doing anything for fifty-three straight hours without sleep, let alone swimming in the ocean under those incredible conditions? Below are quotes from Diana after her amazing swim.

"With all the experience I have, especially in this ocean, I never knew I would suffer the way I did," she said. "For forty-nine hours the wind just blew like heck, and it was rough. It was really rough that first day, Saturday, after the start and I just thought: *Forget about the surface up. Get your hands in somehow, and with your left hand, say, push Cuba back, and push Florida towards you.*" Nyad said through it all, she held her mantra close: You don't like it. It's not going well. Find a way.

"I have three messages," an exhausted and happy Nyad told reporters as she walked onto the beach in Key West. Her face was sunburned and swollen. "One is we should never, ever give up. Two is you never are too old to chase your dreams. Three is it may look like a solitary sport, but it's a team."

By the way, Diana Nyad is sixty-four years old at this writing and has accomplished what no human being in history has ever done. If she can swim 112 miles through the ocean currents and wind non-stop at the age of sixty-four, without a shark cage or wetsuit, you can also reach your goals and dreams if, and only if, you never, ever give up!

Chapter 17

Walking/Running

"The only people who never fail are those who never try."

—*Ilka Chase, American actress and novelist*

Okay, you've decided to start a walking and/or running program as part of your cardiovascular efforts, along with your new low-carb diet plan to lose weight and become physically fit. This will give you more energy, lower your chance of acquiring some types of cancer, heart disease and all the rest of those obesity-related diseases; and you will lose weight. Now how do you start?

First, before you begin any serious exercise program, see your doctor. You know you are overweight and may have additional health issues that are either directly or indirectly caused by being overweight. Tell your doctor what you are planning to do regarding your new exercise program and let him or her check you out and tell you that your plan is fine, based on your present condition. Your doctor may also suggest you opt for a different type of exercise program based on his findings. Assuming your doctor says you can start a serious walking and then running program for your daily cardiovascular activity, the best place to start is with the best walking or running shoes you can afford.

Find the Right Walking Shoes

Go to a store that specializes in selling walking and running shoes. Not the big box sports stores, but a running store. Talk to someone there about your plan so they have as much information as possible about you and what you want to accomplish. This allows them to recommend the best shoe for you, rather than what you see on TV that looks cool. And do not buy serious walking or running shoes for the color, either. Having the right shoe and the right fit for your weight, build, and goals is critical. This makes your walking/running comfortable and reduces the chance of pain or injury from wearing the wrong type of shoe. And believe me, it happens.

The salespeople can also most likely recommend the types of socks to wear and what type of clothes you should wear, depending on the time of year and where you live. These stores will probably have some good books on walking and running as well, and there are hundreds of books on these subjects on the Internet to explore. Checkout amazon.com and type in "walking" or "running" in the search box and see what comes up.

* See Chapter 17 for my walking/running guide to get started.

Laura's Walking-Shoe Research

A while back, I had various issues with my feet, hips, legs, and lower back, and that kept me from effectively doing my hour of daily cardio walking. All this started about six months after my second knee replacement on March 31, 2011.

While I now have two perfectly straight legs after twenty years of limping along on crooked pins, and walking 150 pounds off in spite of this tremendous, weighty handicap, my lower body infrastructure needs some TLC and realignment work. Just like your car.

Meanwhile, as I worked with several of my doctors to get my skeleton straightened, improve my walking, and find my new normal, I decided to get a fresh pair of walking shoes to start off clean without any peculiar wear patterns that could keep me in an incorrect walking rut.

The best advice I can give you to make sure you take that cardio walk in comfort every day is to buy the finest pair of walking shoes you can afford.

And Crocs are *not* walking shoes. That said, here's my personal walking shoe review:

For those of us who need tremendous stability, cushion, and comfort, my hands-down, all-time fave is the Ariel by Brooks. No question. Brooks Beast is the comparable model for you guys out there.

And to find a few other options for you, I polled my good guy pal in Baltimore, Doug Crusse, the Genius marketing director of world-famous Holabird Sports, the largest sporting shoe store in the country. (Their prices can't be beat and they ship second-day air for free!) Here's what he recommended and what I found with each of these shoe styles:

1. The Saucony Grid Omni was just okay and not really anything special compared with my current Brooks Adrenaline and Ariels that I've been wearing since I began walking in earnest in 2003. These babies carried me 35,000 miles, the equivalent of walking around the Earth at the equator about one and a third times. But lately, due to my physical issues, I'm looking for something more— more room in the toe box, for one. And maybe just a little bit more stability and a smoother ride, for another. So, for me, back to the Brook's Ariels for now.

2. The Asics Kyano 17s did not work for me at all. So, don't even bother. Unless you weigh ninety-eight pounds and don't overpronate.

3. I liked the Asics 2160 a lot, but they came in third place of the bunch. Why settle for third when you're really on the hunt for, and deserve, number one?

4. When I tried the Brooks Addiction Walkers and the salesman suggested I try on a bit wider shoe—well, you know how we girls are: At the merest mention of trying on a larger size of anything, we instantly slide into a vanity tailspin. Bigger size? Moi? Wider? What? My feet—still growing? I mean, spreading! None of us gals,

wants to think that our feet are expanding as we—dare I say it—get a bit older. So, I decided to suck it up and get the wider pair. After all, size is only a number, right? Well, turns out the guy knew his stuff and that in my normal, but just a teeny-bit-wider size, the Brooks Addiction Walkers felt like heaven and they were on sale.

5. The New Balance 927s came in a close second to the Brooks Addiction Walkers, but after wearing them around the house for several hours, my feet, legs and back were sore. This model didn't give me the bang for the buck that I was expecting. While comfort always wins out, economics had a heavy hand in my decision, too. Still, if the on-sale Brooks Addiction Walkers didn't really fill the bill the way I needed, I wouldn't have given them a second look no matter what the price.

Our feet support us and carry us everywhere, and we need to take much better care of them than we do. We're gonna be on 'em for the rest of our lives, God willing. When you *think* you're no longer able to change a situation, like your unhealthy, unwanted weight, start by getting an absolutely terrific new pair of walking shoes and get going today. That way, you can challenge yourself to change yourself one step at a time.

Note: As of press time, I jumped ship and went back to Brooks Ariel; that shoe gives the best ride with incredible cushion and the stability's off the charts. And if you overpronate like I tend to, this is the shoe, hands down, that's absolutely right for you. Remember, it's the Brooks Beast for you boys.

Walking Tips

A safety tip: Always tell someone what your usual route is going to be, if you are not on a treadmill indoors, in case there is an emergency and someone needs to reach you. It is a good idea to keep your cell phone with you; many people, especially women who walk or run alone, carry a whistle. Having a walking or running partner increases your chances of success because both of you are now accountable to each other to not skip a day. It's all about reinforcement for success.

And if your dog is your walking partner, so much the better. If you don't have one, borrow one. I could not have developed the daily walking discipline that I did without my two Italian Greyhound walking partners. Got so they craved their daily walks even more than I did and relentlessly bugged me till I gave in and took them for a nice long walk.

Start slow and work your way up. You probably haven't done any distance walking or running in years so don't go crazy on day one. Plan a route for yourself if you are not walking/running on a regular track. Start with a walking plan especially if you want to walk at a brisk pace. Not slow or speed walking, but briskly. For the first few days, you'll want to just walk at a good clip, but not necessarily fast yet, so your muscles can become used to this activity. Then you can start walking even faster. And be sure to stretch those calves and hammies!

Set Your Goals

Your goal is to get your heart rate into that cardio range where it is doing some good. Again, start at what you can comfortably do without killing yourself—start slowly. It won't happen overnight. You want to gradually work your way up to be in the range of about 70% to 80% of your maximum heart rate. There is a rule of thumb of subtracting your age from 220 and multiply that by 70% for your target. You can check your own pulse after you walk or run for a while to see what your heart rate is. You can wear a heart rate monitor on your wrist and check it. So, if you are forty years old, then your target heart rate should be 220 − 40 = 180 x 70% = 126, or 144 at the 80% mark.

Document your progress. It's always good to track your efforts to see where you were when you started your program and how you are progressing. It reinforces your success and efforts to continue and not give up or take a day off from your fitness plan. You can make your own chart or download several samples of walking/running charts off the Internet. The main thing is to write down how far you walked or ran and how much time it took.

Set some achievable goals for yourself and make them happen. Don't get frustrated or discouraged if you don't hit a goal, and never, ever give up. Just keep at it. If you set a goal that was too aggressive, the main thing is to just make progress. A sustainable effort and measurable progress over time will yield results.

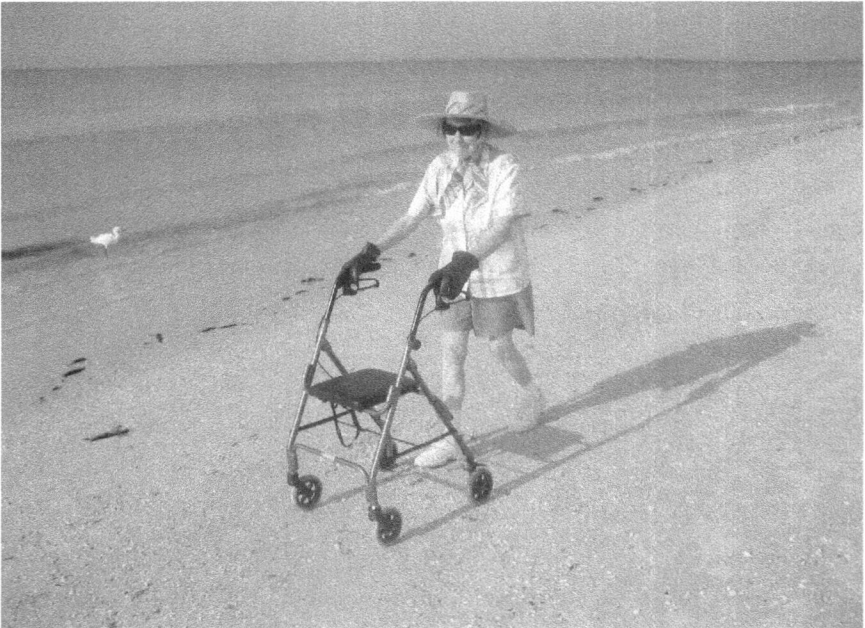

She's walking, isn't she? 87 years old,
walks every day. What's your excuse?

Interval Training

In the past decade, the concept of interval training has become very popular. This is especially true with walking/running and swimming. The idea is to mix up your program with various levels of energy and distance. Interval training keeps your muscles from getting used to just one pace or distance. For beginner walkers, you'll want to try walking at a normal pace for a set distance, maybe a quarter mile, then change to a brisk or very fast walk for one-eighth or a quarter mile, then repeat. You can change the distance and the pace as you wish. When you have progressed to the point that you are just running, you can take the same approach. Slow jog for a certain distance and then change to a fast jog or sprint for a short distance and then back to a slow jog. Introducing a faster pace every once in a while will help you build endurance and strength. Pretty soon, the portions of your training that include a faster pace will get longer and longer and the time and distance you cover will also increase.

Pay Attention to Any Pain

Since you have now started your walking/running fitness program, pay close attention to the reaction and feedback from your body. Of course in the beginning, your muscles will be sore because you haven't been using them. Those first couple of weeks, probably doing this every other day is smart. You don't want any early overexertion injuries or problems from your newfound willpower. After a couple of weeks, you should be able to do this every day. Throughout your fitness program, your muscles will get sore sometimes and that's fine. You just don't want serious pain.

If you are pushing yourself too hard, you may start to feel light-headed. If you feel some pain in your chest, legs, or back, then stop running and walk till you feel better. You've gone too far and your body is letting you know about it. Listen to what your body tells you. Sore is okay, pain is not okay. You do have to suck it up for weight-loss and wellness success, but if you have pain that doesn't go away or if you keep feeling pain when you do something, then go see your doctor and tell him or her everything that you have been doing and get checked out. Don't wait.

So, where is a good place to walk or run? Everywhere except on the street. You may see people jogging along two-lane roads but it is not advisable for safety's sake. You can walk or run at your health club on the treadmill or a running track, if they have one. The treadmill will have more cushion in it than a hard surface if you want to start easy. Find out if your local high school allows community residents to run on the track around the football field. The sidewalks in your neighborhood are fine but if you are walking or running before sunrise or after sunset, wear reflective clothing so cars, motorcycles, and bicycles can see you ahead.

If you can find a very large block, it helps eliminate the boredom of running laps around a smaller block. Many urban areas have large parks to run in, and outside the cities there may be forest preserves where you can run. They usually have an asphalt running/bicycle path that snakes for miles with several entrance or exit points. It makes the time go faster, there are no worries about vehicles, and you're out walking or running in nature.

Twelve-Week Program for Getting to Thirty Minutes of Nonstop Running*

Here is an excellent walk/run program that will allow you to get to the point of being able to run for thirty minutes within three months, courtesy of www.best-running-tips.com, an informative running website. The walking part is at a very brisk pace and not a normal casual pace. The run is at a decent jogging pace.

This is a three day per week program to start. Pick your days with one day of rest in between. After you have completed this and can run for thirty minutes nonstop, you can start increasing your minutes a little each day. Maybe just add five additional minutes for the week per day. So, on week thirteen you will run for thirty-five minutes each day, and in week fourteen you will be at forty minutes per day. If this is too much, then only add three minutes instead of five. Your body will tell you what it can or can't handle.

There are many running clubs across the country to join, get advice from, and participate in races, if you like. If you get really serious about running and enjoy it, there are literally hundreds, if not thousands, of races each year for every ability level and a wide range of distances. There are triathlons, too, if you want to add some distance swimming and biking to your distance running races. The Resources section at the end of this book has many links to websites of interest as well as walking/running magazines, accessories, etc. Now get out there and start putting some serious mileage on those new shoes!

*As with any new diet and fitness plan, be sure to check with your physician before you begin.

Chapter 18

Create Your Own Future—Now

"Depression is the inability to construct a future. "

—Rollo May, American psychologist and author

If Rollo May is right, it's no wonder so many of us become increasingly depressed with our struggles to lose weight. And, is it any wonder that we feel helpless when our health, fitness, and lives are at stake? There's almost nothing I hate more than seeing people grapple needlessly, unnecessarily with their weight.

So, if depression really is the inability to construct a future, then it's time to get busy constructing your own happier, healthier future. You have to have a hand in creating your new health and fitness plan* that you can live with forever, in order for it to work for you. There're lots of other things in life to be depressed about besides certain issues you have total control over, such as your weight, your health, your fitness, and your life.

The American motivational speaker and author, Earl Nightingale, said, "We tend to live up to our expectations." You must start somewhere—and once you do, expect to reach your goals. For what we expect in life tends to happen, one way or another. Start your weight-loss journey by keeping a daily fitness journal, a place to record your progress on the steps you take toward your new, forever lifestyle change.

Weigh Yourself Daily

Next, it is imperative to weigh yourself every day. I cannot stress this enough. You absolutely need to know when you're holding at the same weight for days (or months) on end, or if you're gaining (heaven forbid). Learn to use those numbers on your scale to motivate you, not defeat you. Weigh only once a day and preferably in the morning after you take care of business, if you know what I mean. And if you weigh naked, weigh that way every single day. Always do it the same, then you'll constantly know where you stand. (This is for you guys out there, too. We know y'all weigh naked.)

If you happen to be visiting the doctor on a particular day, note how much you weigh on your scale that morning and then how much you weigh on your doc's scale later. Mark it in your fitness journal beside that morning's weight and note it so you won't freak. You'll be heavier on your doc's scale with clothes on and it'll be later in the day so you'll have had things to drink and eat. Just make a quick note, close your journal and get on with your day. Don't dwell on it and beat yourself up. It's not what you really weigh, anyway—your morning weight is.

In July 2013, the University of North Carolina and UNC Lineberger Cancer Control Education Program Fellowship sponsored a study on how daily self-weighing versus occasional self-weighing affects the weight loss efforts of overweight people. After six months, the results published in Obesity magazine indicated "daily self-weighing can produce clinically significant weight loss."

Steinberg, D. M., Tate, D. F., Bennett, G. G., Ennett, S., Samuel-Hodge, C. and Ward, D. S. (2013), The efficacy of a daily self-weighing weight loss intervention using smart scales and e-mail. Obesity, 21:1789–1797. doi:10.1002/oby.20396

Oprah, who has shed a lot of weight throughout the ages, recently said she "does not want to be a slave to her scale" and she "hasn't weighed herself since January." Excuse me, and with all due respect, but she also has every weight-loss resource, shrink, chef, coach, personal trainer, and guru in the world at her fingertips. She can afford *not* to be a slave to her scale. But you and I can't. Learn to use that number you see between your tootsies every morning as part of your motivation for the day.

Don't look at weighing every day as being a slave to anything other than moving step by step toward mastering your healthier eating and how much you walk. Knowledge is power, so know what you weigh. It's one of the most powerful tools you have to help resist eating things you should not be eating.

Most overweight people's body sense has gone haywire; their body awareness is buried under years of dieting failures and physical neglect. If your life stays the way it is now, so will your weight.

By not weighing myself every day, by "listening to my body's needs," by "trusting my body's awareness," and, my very favorite, "by eating what I need to get along," my butt skyrocketed all the way up to 317 pounds. Never again. I learned my lesson and hope you'll learn from me before it's too late.

One Step at a Time, One Pound at a Time

Take the advice you find in this book to heart; try it, practice it, live it— and you'll knock those excess pounds down, this time for good. Relax and give yourself some time. Take it one step at a time, one pound at a time. Hell, there are times I take it a quarter of a pound at a time. Whatever works, do it. Just walk and weigh every single day and get over it, already. There really is no other way.

Remember, not one of us is overweight because aliens swooped down from the sky, captured us in our sleep, whisked us off to the mother ship and force-fed us milk shakes, pizzas, cookies, popcorn, and cheesecakes before returning us to our beds and unsuspecting families. We all did it to ourselves—some of us knowingly and some of us unwittingly. Either way, it's time to dig our way out of this bottomless pit together and learn to live and enjoy our lives the way we were intended to—healthy, joyfully, gorgeously, and, above all, unencumbered.

Start by

1. Writing down your three top weight-loss and fitness goals and the timeframe in which you will achieve them.

2. Picking your low-carbohydrate lifestyle eating program (i.e., diet).

3. Weighing yourself at the same time every day.

4. Working thirty to sixty (sixty is the goal) minutes of *daily* cardio into your life.

5. Using the following five-week walking and fitness logs to help you stay on track during your crucial first thirty-five days.

6. Refer to Part Five, Laura's Commit-to-Get-Fit TIPS, for motivation, inspiration, Ask Laura letters/responses, and ideas that will keep you on track and working toward your goals.

*As with any new diet and fitness plan, be sure to check with your physician before you begin.

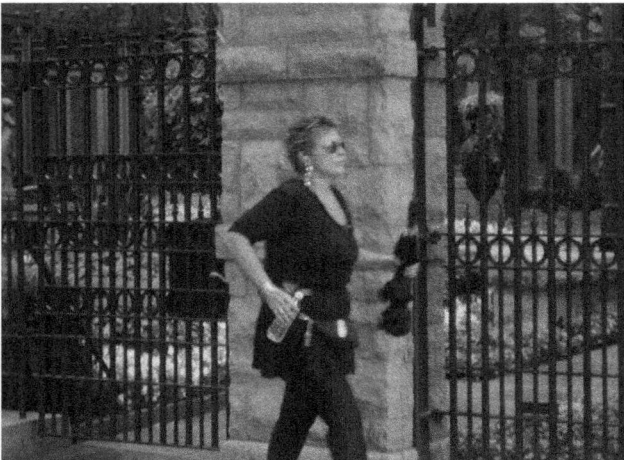

Week 1: Walking and Fitness Log

"In order to attain the impossible, one must attempt the impossible."

—*Miguel De Cervantes, Spanish novelist, dramatist, poet*

All I can tell you is this: until you learn to make walking a daily habit, you will not lose any weight. Diet and daily exercise go hand in hand on the path to better health and fitness. What better exercise is there than walking?

Day and Date	Steps	Miles	Time	Water Consumed	Carbs Consumed	Weight	
Sun							
Mon							
Tue							
Wed							
Thu							
Fri							
Sat							
Total							

What are your health and fitness goals for this week?

What was the high point of your week?

What was the low point?

What's bugging you?

What are you prepared to do about it to make things better and more productive, health- and fitness-wise, next week? And the week after that, and the week after that ...

Week 2: Walking and Fitness Log

"Don't measure yourself by what you have accomplished, but by what you should have accomplished with your ability."

—*John Wooden, American basketball coach*

We all have the ability to be more healthy and fit than we currently are. What we accomplish with that ability is strictly up to us. We can chose to lose weight and get healthy or we can remain the same and probably die way before our time.

Day and Date	Steps	Miles	Time	Water Consumed	Carbs Consumed	Weight	
Sun							
Mon							
Tue							
Wed							
Thu							
Fri							
Sat							
Total							

What are your health and fitness goals for this week?

What was the high point of your week?

What was the low point?

What's bugging you?

What are you prepared to do about it to make things better and more productive, health- and fitness-wise, next week? And the week after that, and the week after that ...

Week 3: Walking and Fitness Log

"Tomorrow's battle is won during today's practice."

—Japanese Proverb

In order to be more healthy and fit tomorrow, you have to begin today. Make daily walking a lifelong practice.

Day and Date	Steps	Miles	Time	Water Consumed	Carbs Consumed	Weight	
Sun							
Mon							
Tue							
Wed							
Thu							
Fri							
Sat							
Total							

What are your health and fitness goals for this week?

What was the high point of your week?

What was the low point?

What's bugging you?

What are you prepared to do about it to make things better and more productive, health- and fitness-wise, next week? And the week after that, and the week after that …

Week 4: Walking and Fitness Log

"Your past is not your potential. In any hour you can choose to liberate the future."

—*Marilyn Ferguson, American writer*

Every day is a new beginning. Put your past behind you. Liberate yourself once and for all. Walk and weigh every day. You can do it—it's not that hard. Staying fat's far more difficult.

Day and Date	Steps	Miles	Time	Water Consumed	Carbs Consumed	Weight	
Sun							
Mon							
Tue							
Wed							
Thu							
Fri							
Sat							
Total							

What are your health and fitness goals for this week?

What was the high point of your week?

What was the low point?

What's bugging you?

What are you prepared to do about it to make things better and more productive, health- and fitness-wise, next week? And the week after that, and the week after that ...

Week 5: Walking and Fitness Log

"Until you value yourself, you will not value your time. Until you value your time, you will not do anything with it."

—*M. Scott Peck, American psychiatrist and inspirational author*

It takes a lot of time and effort to overeat, e-mail jokes, blabber on the phone, and watch TV. Make time everyday to take a walk instead. Notice where you waste time. Do something about it. Value yourself first. If you don't, no one else will.

Day and Date	Steps	Miles	Time	Water Consumed	Carbs Consumed	Weight	
Sun							
Mon							
Tue							
Wed							
Thu							
Fri							
Sat							
Total							

What are your health and fitness goals for this week?

What was the high point of your week?

What was the low point?

What's bugging you?

What are you prepared to do about it to make things better and more productive, health- and fitness-wise, next week? And the week after that, and the week after that …

Part Four

Motivation and Inspiration

Chapter 19

Motivation

"If you want to find out about the road ahead, then ask about it from those coming back."

—*Chinese Proverb*

One very important aspect of motivation is to find the willingness to stop and realistically look at exactly what you're eating and the ways you're behaving that keep your weight on. Then do something about it. This simple process of focusing on foods that you normally take for granted, like what you *think* is healthy eating, is a powerful source for improved health, wellness, happiness, and creativity.

Sooner or later, you're gonna get sick of the yo-yo cycle and just do what it takes to get your weight off and keep it off, once and for all.

Motivation and Self Esteem

Who can tell me what this statement means? *You have to do what you have to do, so you can do what you want to do.*

Self-esteem or lack thereof affects every aspect of our lives. It's how we feel about ourselves and influences how we live our lives. First, you need to love yourself unconditionally. And this is not a cliché: if you don't, who will?

Then you've got to really believe in yourself, no matter what. Believe that this diet, health, and fitness plan* will be the last time you go through this struggle. Convince yourself that, deep down in your bones, you know that you can do it one more time—once and for all.

What does self-esteem mean to you? Self-esteem refers to a person's mental picture of her or himself. It's how you really look at yourself every day. Self-esteem is two things in particular: how others see or treat us, and how we see and treat ourselves. Both have a big impact on our self-esteem.

A lot of our self-esteem is also based on interactions we have with other people and our life experiences. This mental picture we have of ourselves contributes to our self-esteem. Self-esteem is all about how much we feel valued, loved, accepted, and thought well of by others—and how much we actually value, love, accept, and think well of ourselves.

People with healthy self-esteem are able to feel good about themselves, appreciate their own worth, and take pride in their abilities, skills, and accomplishments. People with low self-esteem feel as if no one will like them or accept them or that they can't do well in anything. Or that they're ugly, fat, clumsy, or just don't fit in with the "in" crowd.

Everyone experiences problems with self-esteem at certain times in their lives—especially during our teens when we're figuring out who we are and where we fit in the world. And it carries right on through to adulthood when, sadly, most of us never fully realize our highest self-esteem potential—especially if we're fat or have some other perceived defect.

The best news is that self-esteem is not fixed for life. So if you feel that your self-esteem isn't all it could be, you can improve it. Try the following exercise:

On a piece of paper or an index card, write all the adjectives you can think of to describe yourself, like:

I'm Fabulous! Creative! Gorgeous! Funny! Nice! Loving! Sensational, talented, smart, sexy, powerful, cute, healthy, worthy of love, loveable.

Post this card where you'll see it every single day and make a second copy to carry around in your wallet as a constant reminder when things get a bit low.

The word *No* is one of the most powerful words there is, both in giving and in receiving. Know why? Being told, "No, you can't do it," or "No, that's not meant for you," are very powerful self-esteem busting statements. I know, because I was raised in a house in which that was the "norm" for me. It takes a lot of courage and hard work to overcome that kind of background, but it is possible to reach unimaginable heights when you do.

Just look at all the people in history who were told, "No, you aren't good enough," and then succeeded wildly: President Obama, Michael Jordan, and thousands of other famous and not-so-famous folks like you and me, too. Your life is what you make it and if you're not satisfied with the soup that's in your cup, what're ya willing to do about it?

Then there's the other side of the *No* coin; the boundary-setting *No*.

"No, I won't allow you to treat me that way." "No, I won't be able to do that for you." These are positive *No's* that definitely set healthy boundaries for us. Think of your own examples.

One of the main reasons why I strongly believe in morning meditation is because the way you start your day usually determines how the rest of your day goes. Agree? Disagree?

Power of Daily Meditation

One of the things that helped me the most when I first began losing weight and needed to develop discipline, increase my will-power, and improve my self-esteem was twice daily meditation. It took about a month to kick in, but once I decided that this was it—this was the last time I would ever be this heavy—I began to crave my twice daily meditations. And once I saw improvement in my diet and daily cardio lifestyle, it was too hard to stop.

Start by writing down your goals, hopes, ambitions, and desires for the day. Take five to ten minutes every morning to do this. It will help you throughout your day and life.

Stop reading and write a few of them down right now. Begin to use these morning lists to prioritize the top three things you want to accomplish each day. Be sure to share this with someone you can trust to support you in your new health and fitness lifestyle plans—someone to help hold you accountable. Eventually, you have to become so strong that you will be able to hold yourself accountable to yourself.

Above all, stop thinking negative thoughts about yourself at once. Negative self-talk is one of the most destructive things you can do to sabotage your new lifestyle efforts and yourself.

Stop reading and write down at least three positive things about you; more, if you have time.

One thing to remember is to always strive for accomplishment rather than perfection. Perfection comes with experience. Perfection comes with doing. What are you doing to *Commit To Get Fit?*

Realize that all mistakes are learning opportunities for you to do better or get it right the next time. Sometimes this can be a painful lesson, but you come away much stronger in the long run.

Always be willing to try new things. Learn new skills—a language, art, take up dance.

Write those on the other side of that little index card or piece of paper.

Carry that little card or piece of paper in your purse or pocket and look at it a few times during the day, especially when things might not be going so well, to keep on track. We ALL need reminders about how wonderful and worthy we are …

Visualize accomplishing each and every one of the things you write on that card or piece of paper.

See yourself successful every day.

Meditate on it.

Set daily, weekly, and monthly—semester or yearly—goals that are within your control, not things that are just way too far outside of what you can realistically achieve right now.

Keep planning and working toward your bigger goals by managing your smaller goals. They all add up and will get you where you're going, as long as you keep working at it every single day, in every way.

Because with hard work you can have achievable goals, but you have to work smart, too. So, get organized, and practice this form of writing for a few minutes every morning because it will help you get on that road to success.

And once you do something you have on your list, you'll feel a tremendous sense of accomplishment; you'll feel good about it and your self-worth will skyrocket.

It's just getting started that's the hard part.

Think about this: How many times did Michael Jordan get kicked off his high school basketball team? How many times has a publisher said, "No, we don't like your book?" to a now-famous author. Study famous people's first steps, not their end results.

And don't study only your heroes' end results, either, but your heroes' first steps.

And then, get out of your own way and watch what happens!

Recognize what you can change and what you can't.

If you're unhappy with something about yourself that you can change, then start today. If it's something you can't change, like the color of your skin, your nose, or your height, then start to work toward loving yourself just the way you are. And figure out how to improve the things you don't like, such as your weight.

Set goals. Think about what you'd like to accomplish, then make a plan to do it. Stick with your plan and keep track of your progress. Take pride in your opinions and ideas and don't be afraid to voice them.

Make a contribution. Tutor a student or classmate who's having trouble. Help clean up your yard or your neighborhood, participate in a walkathon for a good cause, or volunteer your time in some way to those less fortunate. Feeling like you're making a difference and that your help is valued can do wonders to improve self-esteem.

Exercise! You'll be healthier and happier and daily exercise relieves stress, and we ALL have stress on us these days.

It's never too late to build healthy, positive self-esteem. In some cases where the emotional hurt is deep or long lasting, it can require the help of a mental health professional, like a counselor or therapist. These experts can act as guides, helping you to learn to love yourself and realize what's unique and special about you.

Self-esteem plays a role in almost everything we do. People with high self-esteem do better on the job, in their careers, and in school and find it easier to make friends. They tend to have better relationships with their younger friends and other adults; feel happier; find it easier to deal with mistakes, disappointments, and failures; and are more likely to stick with something until they succeed.

It takes a little work to develop good self-esteem, but once you do it's a skill you'll have for life. Magic Johnson was asked what makes the difference between winners and losers. He answered: "The difference between winners and the losers is that the winners lose more than the losers—they just keep getting back up, going to practice and giving it their all each time they're on the court! The court of life!"

Do Your Own Research; It's Your Body and Your Life

Obesity and poor health are realities, but they no longer have to be a personal issue for you. Plus, being obese is just plain unhealthy. And unnecessary. And totally preventable. If you don't have a good doctor, or if you're not having satisfactory results with your current doctor, ask around. Call your local hospital for referrals. Interview doctors or their head nurses on the phone and tell them what you have in mind. See where their heads are with regard to low-carb dieting and fitness, especially. Ask what type of weight-loss programs they believe in and what kind of success they're having with other obese patients. Tell them how much weight you want to lose, what you've been doing to get as fat as you are now, and what you'd like to do to get healthier.

If you don't like what you hear, call the next doctor on your list and keep calling until you find one that is right for you. If you're lucky, you'll discover one like I did (Dr. Mark Stolar with Northwestern Internists, Ltd., Chicago). The man never prejudged me just because I was grossly overweight. He listened to everything I had to say and then tested and

worked hard to find out *why* I was having such a difficult time losing weight.

I am often asked what I like most about losing 150 pounds and becoming a totally different-looking person. Besides feeling a whole lot better physically, mentally, and emotionally, it's the power of knowing that for the first time in my life I'm in *total* control.

I control exactly what I eat, how much I move and just

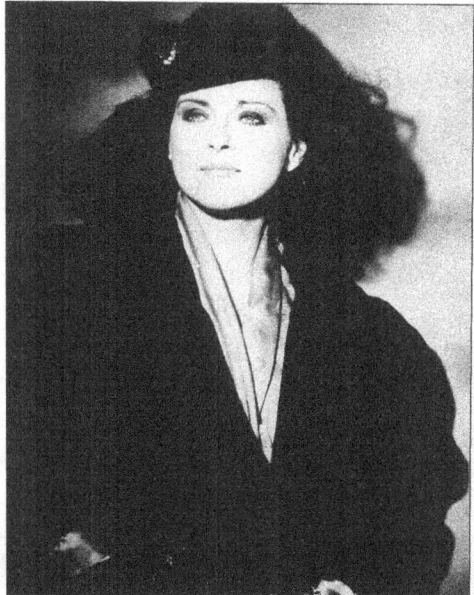

about everything else in my life that I want. I never realized I had this kind of power before. I always knew I was a very strong gal and that I could accomplish just about anything I set my mind to, but being able to control my weight eluded me my entire life—until now. It's beyond my wildest dreams to be able to wield this kind of power, especially over myself. And the more success I have, the more determined and motivated I am to maintain it.

Losing 130 pounds in two and a half years—the old-fashioned way—and then knocking off about twenty more and keeping it off for over ten years is an incredible achievement that has totally changed my life. If I can do it, you can, too. It's not all that difficult. You have to make up your mind that you really want to. I can show you the way, but I can't change your mind for you. No one can. No doctor, shrink, spouse, or partner—no one but you. You gotta wanna.

Figure out what you hate most about being the weight you are right now. You'll find it won't be just one single thing. Make a list and look at it every day. Then do something about it. Find your "Perfect Storm." Use it as motivation.

Never Give Up on Your Dream

If your dream is to be svelte or Speedo-worthy by summer, figure out your own roadblock to getting fit and rid yourself of it. Meditate about it, pray about it, but, whatever you do, take steps to obliterate that obstacle and get your butt moving in a much healthier direction.

Combine your daily cardio practice with a good, healthy, low-carb eating plan* and watch what happens. Your weight will literally melt off like magic, I promise, but you gotta wanna—and you have to be dedicated and diligent in your efforts. You know you can't do anything like this half-assed. You have to be ready to give it your all—and that means you have to make up your mind to begin right now, today, right where you are.

Regardless of what types of food you have in your house, fridge, and hidey-hole, eliminate everything that doesn't support your new health and fitness eating plan. Ditch the oatmeal, cereals, breads, pastas, cookies, and cakes; anything and everything that's too high glycemic, get rid of it. Purge all the rest of those white starch and sugar carbs lurking around and get yourself going. Give it all away, and not to someone who needs to lose a bit of unhealthy, unwanted poundage, either. It's much better to either give these things to friends who can afford to eat them, the ones with a better metabolism than you and I have, or throw them away. You know what will happen if you don't, eventually you'll be wearing it.

Never give up on your dream to be healthier and more fit just because of the time it will take to accomplish it.

Food Is Not Love; Nor Is It Applause

All I can tell you is this: food is not love. I know, I know. Try telling that to your eighty-seven-year old Nonna, who absolutely does not get the concept at all. To her generation, food was love, is love, will always be love, and that's exactly the way they want it. These women showered their families with food-love, keeping them all happy, healthy, well-loved and well-fed—and, in a lot of cases, like mine, fat.

When I first began my latest and last weight-loss and fitness quest, I had to cut out all—and I mean *all*—breads, pastas, sweets, rice, and all other white starchy, sugary, and high-glycemic foods and fruit in order to lose my unhealthy, unwanted weight. As you can see, it didn't kill me. I'm still here and I don't suffer one bit.

However, I do keep a raptor's eye on pretty much everything I eat, especially during the week. I grant myself special dispensation to eat pretty much whatever I want, in reasonable portion sizes, on Saturday (date) nights. But, you can do this only after you reach your target weight loss and wellness goal.

Also, you might consider starting to cut your portion sizes a bit. This is another crucial key to true and everlasting weight loss, besides weaning yourself off those white, starchy, sugary carbs. This way, if you can't quit the carbs cold turkey, at least you'll be headed in the right direction. It took me a good ten days to two weeks to wean myself off all the carbs that were hurting me. And that's exactly what you do when you choose to stay fat: you hurt yourself repeatedly.

Do what you have to do to stop eating that sweet, starchy, white junk. If you don't eat it, you won't crave it. Simple as that. That's why a low-carb lifestyle diet like the Atkins Diet, The Zone Diet, and South Beach Diet* work well for me and others just like me. I assure you, once you break your carb addiction and work to keep it broken, the easier your weight loss will be.

If I knew when I was younger what I know now about white, starchy, sugary carbs being deadly for me, and about the extreme importance of daily cardio/fitness walking to lose weight and then keep it off forever, I never would have spent a lifetime being fat. But we didn't know then what we know now.

And for those of you who're looking for more applause: learn to sing, dance, paint, write, act, or learn to eat right. What a novel thought! Stop the weekly baking for your family's and co-workers' applause. You're enabling them and yourself with your baking.

The problem is that we're led to believe all those homemade goodies in front of us were made especially for us with tender love, sweat, and care, so it confuses us into thinking that food **is** love. I've been there; food really isn't love.

Baking is actually one of the biggest downfalls with people regaining their weight, believe it or not, for both the baker and for the bake-ees—the eaters of all those homemade goodies. I've seen it happen time after time after time. And most would rather have the applause than a thinner, lighter, healthier body. Can you believe that? Don't let it be you. And all those yummy desserts you bake for your co-workers' applause? They're your biggest downfall. The bananas you use in your award-winning banana bread are poison for a low-carb diet—and to anyone that overproduces insulin, like you, like me. And I know you eat those dang 'nanners because you always mention them so lovingly when we talk.

When someone's weight loss is stalled or on the uptick, it's always due to what they're eating, and a lot of the time it's due to their baking. Seriously. Or due to others' baking: "I made this especially for you!"

And here's the excuse: I'm the baker at work; everyone counts on me to bring my home-baked goodies every week. What would they all do without my homemade treats? The more important question is this: what would you do without all that applause? Because that's really why you bake for the office, your family, and your church group or gathering in the first place.

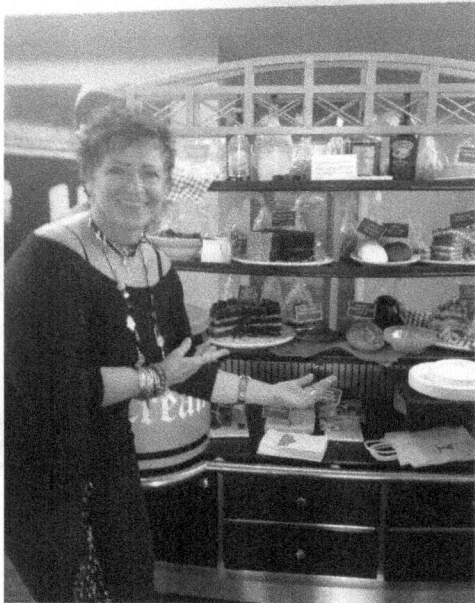

We've all done it, we've all been there, and some of us are stalled there right now, and I'd say addicted to the applause besides the carbs, too. Get over it. Either learn to make your recipes healthier and low-carb using natural sweeteners and alternative flours and such, or find new recipes that lend themselves to your diet, health, and fitness plan. And keep your mouth shut about it until people begin to compliment you on your new recipes … then 'fess up, if you want to. What they don't know won't hurt them. And if you make your recipes low carb and healthier, you'll really be helping them!

Whatever you do, please stop baking the way you're doing it now. You'll never lose your unhealthy weight if you don't.

I wish you could hear the lame excuses people use far too often when their weight isn't coming off the way it should, given the amount of effort they claim they're putting in; you kids can't fool me. I've lived a lifetime right where you are now. I know exactly what I ate to be 317 pounds and I know exactly what you're eating and not doing in the way of daily cardio to keep yourself fat.

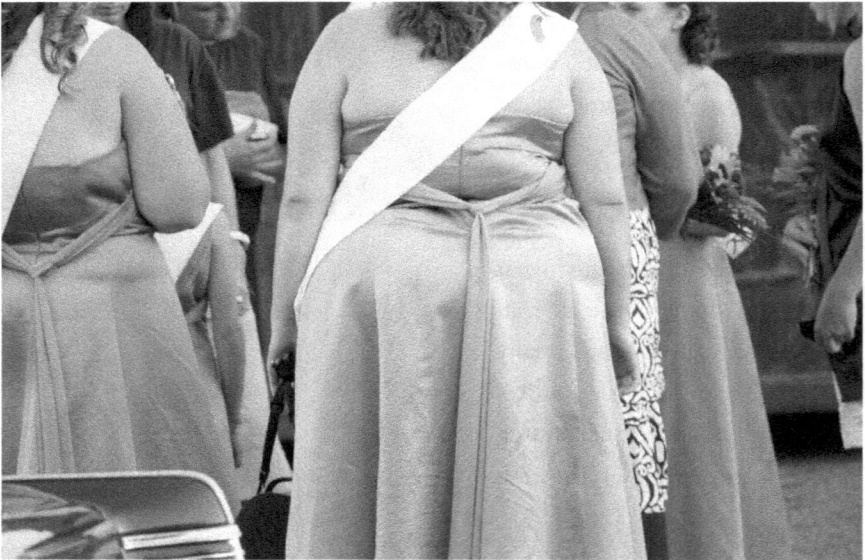

It's not love, it's just food, and if the temptation is too great, you have to get it out of your house. Give it away to some poor, deserving soul who doesn't have anyone else making them such homemade goodies. Share the wealth with your neighbor, Pilates instructor, doorman, hairdresser, janitor, parking attendant, teacher, librarian, whomever you think would appreciate and enjoy all that "love" on a plate.

And don't let the guilt of not eating all that "love" get you down. Look at it as a step in a better, much healthier direction.

I wrestle with temptation all the time. I'm hit on a daily basis with thoughts of eating certain foods and sweets that I shouldn't. But, like a lot of other people who want to overcome some sort of addiction, I deal with it. When I put my hands on that cookie, when I'm offered that scrumptious piece of pie or candy, I have to tell myself *no*: capital N, capital O.

There is no other way. It's called personal responsibility.

And then as fast as you can say, "Hot Fudge!" my life flashes right before my eyes, reminding me how much easier it is to get around, how much better I feel, how much better I look now that I weigh 150 pounds less.

Use whatever psychological weapons and tricks you have at your disposal to overcome the urge to eat whatever you want, especially when you know it's not good for your new diet lifestyle plan. "Just a taste" of the wrong thing at the wrong time will set you back, so why tempt fate? Why play into your demon's hands? Remember: The first bite always tastes as good as the last, so why do you need to eat the whole thing?

And if you're just beginning your new health and fitness plan,* this is the wrong time to be tasting any forbidden foods. Make sure you get done what you need to get done in the way of diet and exercise to move successfully through each day.

Not So Easy

The following is by Ralph Marston, author of *The Daily Motivator*. "It is easy to do nothing. Yet what is easiest is not always the best. It is easy to hope for the best outcome. To actually bring it about often requires difficult and even painful decisions, actions, and solid, tangible commitment.

"It is easy to criticize the actions of others, particularly in hindsight, or to speculate about what should have been done. But nothing ever has been accomplished by criticism or speculation alone. Accomplishment comes from those who are willing to put themselves on the line. The world moves forward because of those people who step up to do what is right and what is best, rather than just what is easiest.

"Taking the easy way out can often lead to results that are not so easy to handle. Doing nothing is easy to justify and easy to implement, but in the long run it ends up being a difficult, burdensome way to live. Make your choices based not on what is easy, but on what is best, and do what you know needs to be done. That's the strategy to take you where you truly would like to be."

*As with any new diet and fitness plan, be sure to check with your physician before you begin.

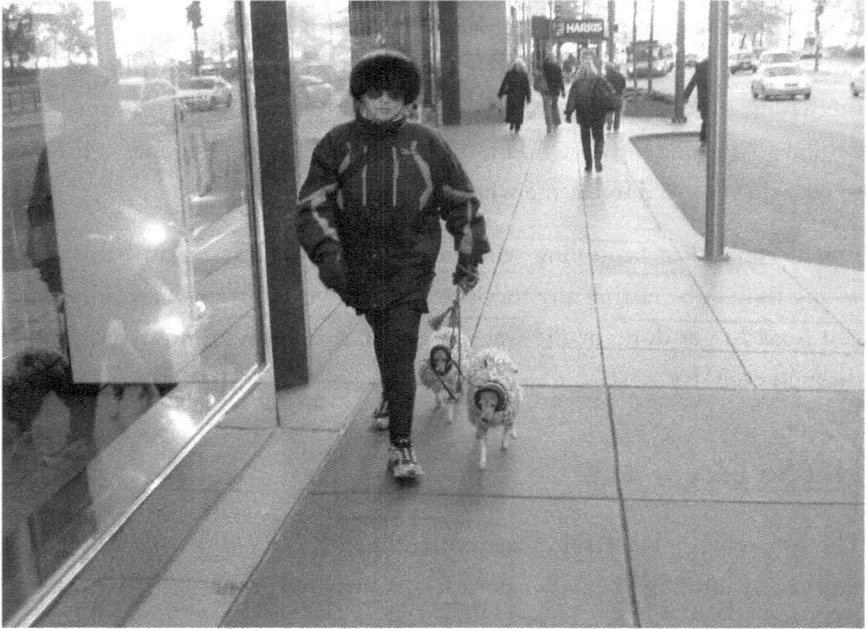

Chapter 20

Inspiration

"The best revenge is massive success."

—Frank Sinatra, American singer and centertainer

How do you want to spend the rest of your life? *Hope* is essential for making any lifestyle change your successful new reality. "Hope is a good thing, maybe the best of things, and no good thing ever dies," according to Andy Dufresne, the character played by Tim Robbins, who was falsely accused of murdering his wife in *The Shawshank Redemption.* He would know. Look what hope did for him.

Hope is a good thing for you, too. With each positive, healthy step you take in the right direction, you'll feel less reluctant and more hopeful on your journey to weight loss and wellness success. With every successful step you take comes more success. Success always breeds success.

Maintaining Your New Lifestyle

You gotta have hope. And determination. And discipline. And you have to have the will to overcome all obstacles that stand before you, whether it's your spouse, significant other, family, friends, boss, or foe. You have to hope that *this time, this diet* will be the last diet for you. This time you will make it to the finish line of weight loss and wellness success. Then the rest is up to you to maintain your new lifestyle forever.

To help remind me of my mission, I even go so far as to tape little notes to places where I might turn for food distraction in a weak moment, like my fridge or freezer, to name two. "Think before you eat it!" "Count those carbs!" "Suicide by Sugar!" and "Eat fewer carbs!" are four of my favorites.

Just ask some of my friends. They think I'm nuts for doing this and always laugh when they see my notes of encouragement, especially after all this time. But what they don't realize is that we all need constant, positive reinforcement and the laugh really is on them. Because they know full well that everything I do to lose and maintain my new weight works.

And if someone brings me carb-laden treats, I thank them and then generally give them away or store them out of reach, far away from the kitchen, in my back storeroom high up on a shelf or in the extra freezer. Stash the stuff anywhere but not right under your nose. Make yourself work to get at it. Gives you time to think and reason with yourself about why you absolutely should not be eating it. Works like a charm for me.

Someone once said, "Change is a process, not a destination." Your destination is reaching a healthy, new goal weight and then keeping it there for life. The process required is not that hard, trust me. Staying fat is way more difficult, takes a lot more energy, requires a good amount of deceit and denial, and involves quite a bit more sacrifice, discomfort, and unhappiness.

Lots of positive, healthy little steps add up to big, lifelong changes. So, have the hope, courage, determination, and the will to become the person you believe you were always meant to be.

Always Do the Right Thing

One day, it was already 11:00 a.m. before I knew what hit me. I had to get out the door to do my cardio before another second passed. I hate when that happens, don't you? It's hard enough to get it in everyday, let alone having to do it quite a bit later than I like. For one minute, I deliriously thought, *Too late to do my daily cardio today! Yippee!*

Then my conscience got the better of me and said, "Have I got news for you, sister; don't even think about not doing it!"

It doesn't matter how long it takes me to get out that door every morning to squeeze in my daily cardio, weights, and physical therapy, I know I have to always do the right thing and get 'er done—no matter what—or I'll suffer physically. And after all my preaching, I hope you're on your way to developing the daily walking health habit for yourself, too. Daily cardio is *that* important to our future health and fitness survival. Seriously.

> One recent weekend, I ran into an avid reader of my weekly motivational articles/blog posts, who told me, and I quote: "Your issues are my issues—and my issues are yours—even though my issues are not necessarily with my weight." This gal is as fit and trim as they come, but I do understand that everyone, no matter what their physical ability, shape, or size, has trouble getting her butt in gear from time to time.

> "I wonder how many of your radio show listeners and column readers realize that your articles are really about motivation, about empowerment, about developing discipline and increasing self-esteem? You're a wonderful role model and catalyst who gives people the impetus and the motivation to do anything at all, and you disguise it as weight-loss and wellness advice."

She continued: "You really make me think about what I'm doing and need to be doing in a day. I know I can always count on you for that extra little push to get me going, whether it be for work, personal, or health-related issues. I know that if I need to complete a project, send in that report, take a power walk, cook a special meal for my family—no matter what, I look to you for the motivation to move forward, especially when I don't want to."

So, kids, when you find yourself in a moment of decision—or indecision—when you've got something that needs to get done and you absolutely don't want to do it (like your daily cardio), deep down, you know the right thing to do, because the very worst thing you can do is nothing at all.

Going the Distance

In August, 1987, I was the very last person to complete the Chicago Triathlon; I made it in four hours and fifty-one minutes. I hope reading the following account of the day's events, which appeared in a 1988 issue of *Big Beautiful Woman* magazine, inspires you to find the motivation to improve everything in your life that needs improving, especially getting healthier and more fit. The entire experience gave me incredible strength, because I found out that the key to success in all things truly is mental.

On the day before the race, all of the contestants had to report to a downtown Chicago hotel with our bikes, helmets, and entrance forms in tow. I quickly learned how to maneuver a ten-speed bike up and down crowded escalators and in and out of elevators with finesse and style. Next came the race clinics, which gave tons of tips to help us get through the next day. But none of the anticipation and preliminary preparation even came close to actually doing the real thing—although every day for over a year I either swam or race-walked for a full hour in preparation, so I thought I was more than ready.

5:30 a.m., race day: I reported in to be body-marked. With a black waterproof marker, they wrote my ID in three-inch numbers that reached from my shoulder to well past my elbow. I was "2541" on both arms. Not to worry, they assured me it would come off. My question was, *when?* I looked like a biker chick from hell.

From there, I proceeded to hang my bike, helmet, towel, Walkman (this was 1987, remember), sunscreen, shoes, shorts, and lipstick (you know me, ever the glamour girl), in a designated area at Olive Park at the end of the one-mile swim portion of the event. I carefully took note where I left my things so I could locate the spot quickly among the 3,999 other bikes already stored there.

My triathlon suit was a stylish purple unitard—the kind you dance in. It wasn't insulated like a Body Glove, because I didn't know I needed one, and they also didn't make them in my size at the time, anyway. Oh, how I wish I had one, though, because one of the most brutal experiences of the triathlon was the one-mile swim from Oak Street Beach to Navy Pier in 59° water, bucking one-to three foot waves. Yes, it took me an hour to swim that course, while I normally do a mile and a half in an hour in my club's pool.

It was quite an inner conflict for me walking the mile to Oak Street Beach in that purple unitard. No towel to hide my butt behind, no shorts to camouflage my hips—only a swim card, determination, and, oh, yeah, goggles, to keep my eyeballs from freezing right out of my head in the icy water.

What the hell, I told myself, *if they don't like how I look, that's their problem.* I strutted my stuff and held my head high, trying not to look too scared. There were 3,999 hard-core triathletes there, and not a flabby one in the bunch. I was the fattest person within a mile radius. Seriously.

The men were great, they all wished me luck and gave me encouragement galore. Thin women just stared; many were downright hostile. Others were in awe. And I confess to some enormous feelings of self-doubt along the way. Did I say, "some?" *WTF was I even thinking when I registered for this thing?*

All of this nonsense was quickly forgotten as soon as I took the plunge. The freezing cold water blew my mind; it was beyond comprehension. I couldn't draw a decent breath. I had to keep changing strokes to breathe and thought I was going to die in Lake Michigan's frigid waters right then and there. The cold, the current, the crowd of swimmers, the waves, and everything going on inside my head—all the fear and frustration, drive and determination, and my anger at all those things made me realize I had to complete this challenge, no matter what. I couldn't turn back even if I wanted to; I was in way too deep to quit.

Suddenly, I found myself fuming. My life as I knew it was in shambles, my marriage was disintegrating; my plus-size clothing design business was just getting off the ground, and a lot of people had made no bones about their expectations of my failure. If I wimped out now, how could I ever trust myself to tackle the other things in life that faced me? How could I be strong, take the type of rejection that comes with building a new company from scratch, the rejection that comes with just "putting it out there" day after day? There was no way I would quit. Not now. Not ever.

One hour and one mile later, I staggered out of the water, exhausted but exhilarated. I decided not to stress myself too much more, so I took my time getting to my bike and belongings. I'm built for comfort, not speed, anyway. And while I might not be the fastest, I sure was steady and with one-third of the triathlon down, I told myself that I had only two-thirds left to go.

The twenty-five-mile bike ride was pretty tough in the blistering sun, 100% humidity, and 98° heat; I admit I thought about quitting a million times. I also could have cheated, as I saw some others do, by choosing to ride only half the course. But I figured that was no way to build character, so, sweating bullets, zipping along on my bike, grinding my teeth, I took all my frustrations and anger out on Lake Shore Drive's pavement, and I'm proud to say I finished that part of the course—my way.

Imagine for a minute what it felt like riding along Chicago's beautiful lakefront on a sweltering-hot summer day with half the traffic lanes on Lake Shore Drive blocked off in one direction for us triathletes and the other half bumper-to-bumper traffic. Motorists and passengers alike must have wondered who this crazy-big woman in the purple unitard and black shorts was, cruising along on her bike all by herself like she didn't have a care in the world—totally making their lives miserable.

I laughed and cried at the same time. Here I was, desolate because my marriage was over, yet delirious with joy because if I could complete this Herculean task set before me, I could accomplish anything. I really felt that I could and would be able to do most everything I put my mind to. Somehow this race had become the ultimate test of my guts.

The next thing I knew, I was parking my bike on lower Randolph Street under the Standard Oil Building (in 1987, it's now AON) and starting on the 6.2 mile run. That's when I knew I had it licked. One skinny woman, who had already finished her run, hissed, "Just starting your run?" It was then I realized I was the last one—the very last one.

"Here she comes folks, the last one—give her a hand!"

"Way to go, purple," one guy yelled, thumbs up in the air. The volunteers sprayed me with water as I race-walked by, keeping time with the music on my Walkman. It wasn't easy to keep going, but by then, it would have hurt too much to stop. Every muscle, every bone, every tendon ached and burned. All I could do was keep moving.

At about the halfway point, I asked one of the workers how much farther to the halfway point and she said, "Just turn around here and save yourself a half mile, no one will know."

"I didn't come all this way to cheat," I told her. "I'd know." But, of course, she couldn't understand. I needed to finish what I started for a complete victory; I needed the accomplishment of knowing that I did the whole darn thing.

I asked one volunteer, as I passed, to call the finish line and make sure someone was there to record my time. I had paid my money, went the distance, and I wanted an official time. When I finally crossed the finish line, only about ten people were left, taking down flags, putting things away for next year's race, but the official timer was there to sign my race bib and record my time. It was like a seal of approval for me.

That day, I saw people who did the triathlon in relay teams of three—one for each event. Others, much thinner and more fit than I, dropped out right before my eyes along the way. But I finished. I went the distance. I made it all the way to the end, and I've never had such an exhilarating experience in my life.

I like to think I competed in that remarkable race for all the plus-size gals and guys out there, who grew up like me, thinking we had some defect or some unacceptable flaw. What I proved by finishing—to myself, anyway— is that you don't have to be thin or a raving beauty to succeed in life. You must simply have the determination, the drive, and the dream to go the distance.

It's all mental.

Use It or Lose It

Not long ago, sitting at a table at a favorite Florida restaurant on the Gulf, we took in the panoramic view of Sanibel Island off in the distance just in time to catch the last half hour of sun gloriously setting on the breathtaking horizon. A handsome, elderly couple sat at the table next to ours. And as the wife gazed longingly out the window at the parade of sunset walkers strolling up and down the water's edge, I overheard some of the couple's conversation. Here's what I gathered:

"I never should have stopped," she sighed. (I knew exactly what she was referring to: the walking.)

"I would give anything to be able to do that again," she continued.

"You could do it, if you tried," comforted the husband. "Start out slow."

"I never should've stopped after my last heart attack. I should've gotten right back into it as soon as I felt better. I never made the effort or took the time. Deep down I knew I was just being lazy and putting every stinking, little thing I could think of first. Now look. I'm lucky I can walk to and from the car. What I wouldn't give to be out there with the rest of them and have that spring in my step once again."

I didn't have to ask any questions or pry; I knew all too well what she was talking about. Many people of all ages seek my help, eager to benefit from my motivational "magic," and a lot of their stories are the same. I hear the words, "I never should've stopped," over and over again. "I got cocky and thought I'd feel fabulous forever. And when I began not to, it required an even greater effort for me to start up again, so I gave up."

It seems the old adage, "Use it or lose it," applies to much more than our libido. It affects everything in life. And the older we get, the more important it is to maintain a good level of physical activity, with walking being the number-one most important thing we can do to improve our health and to lengthen our lives.

It's essential to keep moving for as long as we're on this great planet. Not a day goes by that I don't pray and meditate for continued mobility, to be gifted with ambulation, no matter what it takes, right up until it's time for me to move into the next plane.

Since I began my daily walking program in earnest on January 1, 2003, I have come to realize just how incredibly important walking and being able to get around and do everything for oneself truly is. Actually, it's what drove me to begin walking in the first place. That, and the fact that I needed an effective form of daily cardio to blast my excess pounds off and keep them off forever. And what better cardio is there than walking? Seriously. We have to walk to get everywhere in life, otherwise life will pass us by.

Anyone who is able to make daily walking a part of their forever lifestyle is way ahead of every diet and fitness game there is. When you develop the habit of daily walking, eventually building up to a minimum of five miles per day, your weight—combined with a healthy, effective diet—will literally melt right off. I'm living proof.

Begin at the beginning. Start slow if you have to, but get your butt out there and do it every dang day. At first, it's not the time or distance that counts, but that you make the effort to walk daily. After about thirty-five straight days, daily walking will become a lifelong healthy habit. But you gotta work it—for it to work for you.

A Good Plan

Even I need a plan, and I know I have to stick to it. Remember: old habits die hard. When you're an addict, your addiction follows you everywhere. My sugar addiction is no exception.

My stomach's been on strike for several weeks due to a couple Saturday night splurges in a row—you know, the ones where you allow yourself to semi-let 'er rip because you've been towing the line for a few weeks with regard to your diet and daily cardio, and are seeing good results, so you figure you're due a nice, big, fat "reward" for your diligence.

Well, my reward was falling face first into a platter full of scrumptious mini cream puffs at a Film Fest after-party—right in front of hundreds of people, but I hoped not too many were aware. And there were mini cannolis with chocolate-dipped ends piled high around the outside edge of that sweet cream puff platter, too. The scrumptious mini cream puffs were mounded in the center of the plate like a volcano, drizzled with a thin thread of chocolate sauce dripping down the sides to a pool on the bottom layer of the puffs. I was helpless. I thought, *My God, it's Saturday night and an after-party, after all.*

By the time I came to my senses, I figure I'd eaten about eight of those little devils. My friend, Clare, came to my rescue and saved me from myself by eating one of the cannolis I stashed on a plate under the flower arrangement on our table.

Why did I do it? I figured, just like most of us do, that since I've been so stellar health and fitness-wise, I deserved a prize. But when you indulge in a bit more carbs than you should, by the time you get a hold of yourself, the damage is usually already done.

Tread lightly, kids. Once you start to reach some of your smaller interim diet goals, it's really easy to get off track; all it usually takes is one full-blown episode or overindulgence of whatever your food or drink addiction is, to set you back eons, if you let it.

Take it from me, tempting as it is, most of the time that bit of food or drink ain't worth it. Remember: redemption comes with your very next meal. Plan to get back on your plan. And the next day, you gotta get right back on that scale to remind yourself where you're going. Use the number you see there, staring at you from between your toes, as motivation.

Renew your resolve; there is no other way. A good plan today is better than no plan for tomorrow. Don't fall into that trap. You gotta have a plan—for today, for tomorrow, for always.

You have it all in you. You know this. I just help coax it to the surface. A good plan today is always better than a perfect plan tomorrow. And if you don't knock that weight off, tomorrow might never come. Make a good plan for today.

*As with any new diet and fitness plan, be sure to check with your physician before you begin.

Part Five

Laura's Commit-to-Get-Fit TIPS

Chapter 21

Weight-Loss and Fitness TIPS

"If you do what you've always done, you'll get what you've always gotten."

—*Anthony Robbins, American life coach,*
self-help author, and motivational speaker

For Safety

- Tell someone where you're going to be walking and when you'll be back.

- Always have a midpoint destination—just in case.

- Develop interesting, safe walking routes and vary them often, if possible.

- Never leave home without your cell phone, ID, money, and pepper spray.

Apparel and Equipment

- Purchase the best walking (or running) shoes you can afford.

- Dress for the weather; always dress as if it were ten degrees warmer than it is.

- Wear layers and moisture-wicking clothing closest to your skin.

- If you're comfy, you're more likely to enjoy your walk and to get out and do it every day.

Plan

- Just get out and walk.

- Start at a comfortable pace and go a short distance.

- Gradually build your distance and speed.

- Stay hydrated—drink lots of water.

- Do something every day to develop the daily walking habit.

Make It Fun

- Listen to your favorite music in one ear as you walk—whatever puts you in a good mood and peps your step.

- Smile big.

- Take your dog along or borrow one.

- Encourage a friend to walk with you.

Keep Motivated

- Walk every day for thirty-five days straight to develop the habit, then keep it going.

- Keep a daily walking journal: Record your steps, miles, and weight, and chart your daily progress.

- Weigh yourself every day and use the numbers on the scale to motivate yourself, *not* to defeat yourself.

Laura's Favorite, Tried-and-True, Healthy Eating Survival TIPS for Holidays, Birthdays, and Beyond

Events with lots of food and drink are always challenging and sometimes can trigger a backslide. Don't let yourself get seduced by your favorite foods and drinks. It's so not worth it. Eat them in total moderation, when you have to. Holidays and special events are just excuses to keep eating more, to keep wallowing in the same old behavior that got you in trouble in the first place. The following are some tips to help you remain in your new, healthful lifestyle.

1. *Bring a drink you really enjoy.* I believe if you're going to fill up on anything, make it something you really enjoy that legally fits your new lifestyle diet plan. When going to a special event where food will be served, and if you have to, bring your own, nurse it, and use it as your drink of choice for the evening. I drink club soda—a fresh, crisp, gassy one—but my all-time evening favorite is a decaf café latte. Invite me over and I show up with both. Drink a big glass of water right before you go to a party or an event featuring food. You'll be glad you did.

2. *Stay away from alcohol if you really want to lose weight.* Ditch the alcohol, kids. You don't need the carbs. Stick with water, or other zero-carb, non-caloric, non-alcoholic beverages. Most alcohol might be low carb but it's the overproduction of insulin that's making you fat, and alcohol is sure to spike your insulin and mess with your metabolism. If you must indulge, make your wine a weak spritzer instead of straight. When I was fat, I was a notorious eggnog freak. I could drink my body weight in the stuff. Now, it's totally out of the question. Eggnog, or any nog for that matter, is loaded with sugar. So what if it's low fat? I never counted a fat gram or calorie to lose any of my 150 pounds, nor to keep them off this long—ever. I only count white starch and sugar carbs, and control portions, period.

3. ***Remind yourself that "low fat" isn't "low carb."*** And if you struggle with one diet after another, I venture to say you're highly insulin resistant and carb sensitive, like me. It's not the dietary fat that makes you fat, it's the carbs. Carbs create overproduction of insulin. Insulin is the fat hormone. Too much insulin keeps you fat, not dietary fat. Ask Dr. Mark Stolar (Northwestern Internists, Ltd., Chicago, IL) or another good endocrinologist, who understands and believes in the healthy, low-carb way of life. He'll set you straight.

4. ***Utilize the "taste-and-toss" technique.*** If you're absolutely dying for something that's one of your traditional all-time favorite foods, especially at cocktail time, take a big bite, chew slowly to savor it, and covertly slip the rest in the garbage. We don't want to hurt the hostess's feelings, but we certainly don't want those nasty carbs clinging to our faces, butts, and other body parts, either. Remember, you wear what you eat.

5. ***Always offer to bring something to the party or event.*** This nicety also helps you control what you eat. If you're eating low carb, bring your favorite low-carb dish or dishes. Leave nothing to chance.

6. ***Ask for a small plate and fork, if only cocktail napkins are visible.*** Skip the scoopers and other chips that dip—they're too high in white, starchy carbs. A friend of mine usually only provides napkins with her appetizers, no plates and forks, so I always ask for a small plate. Respectfully, I heap it up with all the low-carb dips and goodies offered, because it's the chips and scoopers that are usually the high-carb culprits. Then I eat all the low-carb goop with a fork, tossing in some celery, broccoli, and cauliflower for crunch. Believe me, your brain really won't know the difference and you won't gain weight.

7. ***Stay away from the carrots on the crudités tray.*** They're too high glycemic, meaning they are too high in starch and sugar; if you

overproduce insulin, they'll retard your weight loss. Celery, cucumbers, cauliflower, and broccoli are better for you. Trust me.

8. *Don't overindulge beforehand; save room for the main event.* At a big dinner, go easy and stop at one heaping spoonful. And if it's your very favorite, well, take two, but that's it. No second plates; one stacked should do ya. It has to. And eat slowly. Savor it. Enjoy it. That said, I'd seriously think about what I can't live without, such as Aunt Tillie's garlic smashed potatoes or Gramma's corn bread stuffing, and adjust your portions accordingly. For me, personally, it's sweet potato casserole in any form as long as it's swimming in butter and sumptuous brown-sugar sweetness. And the desserts.

9. *Keep away from the sweets table.* This is the most difficult one for me. I'm a true sweet-a-holic and that's usually the first place I gravitate toward on my initial gastronomic recon mission. My motto used to be: "Life is short, eat dessert first." Well, no more! I finally learned my fat lessons well, and now know when to say "no." I always tell people that I firmly believe I'm only one really good Ghirardelli hot fudge-brownie sundae away from 317 pounds and climbing—and it's no joke.

10. *Think before you eat it.* Do I really need all those white starches and sugary carbs? Remember, they're poison for a person who is carb sensitive and needs to lose weight. If you are overweight, and struggle with one diet after another, that's probably you. For us food junkies, sadly, our addiction's written all over our faces and bodies, unlike alcoholics and drug addicts, who have a much easier time hiding their habit.

11. *Remove yourself from the buffet area ASAP.* Join a group that is having vigorous verbal stimulation or start your own interesting, lively topic of conversation.

12. ***Offer to help the hostess.*** Pick up plates, serve drinks, do whatever. Keep moving and not stuffing yourself. Keep busy and out of the food. Get up and clear the table. Tidy up the dishes. Take out the garbage. Just move.

13. ***Host your own party (holiday, birthday, or any special day) so you can control all of it.*** Make sure you have plenty of tasty low-carb appetizers, beverages, salads, and sides on hand.

14. ***Get out and walk after the big meal.*** Do the dishes for the hostess/host, then drag her/him out with you. Most will welcome the walk, the help, and the fresh air. Always bear in mind: you cannot exercise away a bad diet, but taking that walk after a holiday, birthday or special celebratory meal will certainly help keep the extra pounds at bay.

15. ***If and when you slip up, immediately cease and desist.*** Do *not* use the excuse, "What the hell, might as well finish off that last piece of pecan praline pie and smother it in real whipped cream, while I'm at it. How much worse can things get at this point?" If you get carried away with what you're eating, don't beat yourself up. Begin again at the very next meal. If you find that you can't help yourself and you're eating like you're gonna be shot at sunrise, well, I can't help ya there—you've been forewarned.

Laura's Lifestyle TIPS

1. ***Learn to meditate.*** If you think you can reach your goals alone, think again. Daily positive self-talk works wonders, but there's also nothing like daily meditation for reinforcing your resolve. Works wonders for me. If it's hard to meditate on your own, find a local meditation group to keep you on track. Or see www.wildmind.org/ in the Resources section.

2. *Remember your personal mantra:* Eat less carbs; do more daily cardio. One hour a day. Minimum. Every day.

3. *Do yourself a favor and buy a pedometer.* A pedometer is an invaluable little gadget for keeping track of how many steps you've taken. That pint-size pedometer keeps me on target with my daily walking. I look forward to that sense of accomplishment I get at the end of each day when I see how many steps and miles I logged. Come Saturday, when I add up all my daily totals for the week, the feeling of achievement multiplies. It's always a big thrill to see how the weeks stack up against one another, how my performance improves, and how those numbers help to keep me motivated. I still walk an average of thirty-eight to fifty-eight miles every week. My personal best was about fifty-nine miles in one week. Please see the Resources section for more information on Digi-Walker, FitBit and JawBone's new UP fitness and cardio tracking devices.

4. *Organize your environment to make your new lifestyle change easier to manage.* Tweaking your fridge, cabinets, pantry, purse, car, briefcase, locker, hidey-hole, and workplace will help you stay on track. Remove all temptation from the fridge, or put the stuff in places where you can't see it as soon as you open the door. Out of sight is usually safely out of mind. If you don't lose your unhealthy weight sooner than later, you will continue to be out of your mindwith endless discomfort, illness, and more. Stock up on all your fave, low-carb foods and snacks and arrange them right smack where you can see them as soon as you open the fridge or cabinet.

5. *A good dose of daily cardio curbs your cravings* so you'll eat less carb-laden crap. A minimum of an hour of daily cardio combined with a healthy, effective low-carb diet spares you from the evils of a lifetime of chronic obesity—and worse.

6. *Stay out of the break room,* if that's where all the Dunkin' Donuts and other harmful carb-y baked goods reside. Just because no one

sees when you sneak in there a few times too many on your way to and from the loo, your pancreas knows it and shows it on your body: you wear everything you eat.

7. *Visualize your new wardrobe, and think of all the compliments you'll get.* How long has it been since you've received compliments on the way you look? If you can visualize a new you, you can create a new you.

8. *Set daily and weekly weight and fitness goals,* but be sure to weigh yourself every day and keep a record of it in your fitness journal. How else will you know where you're going if you don't keep a daily health and fitness journal? It's your roadmap to success. Use your morning weight to motivate yourself. Writing down how far and how long you walk, and how much you weigh every single day will also help motivate you to gradually accomplish doing more, pushing yourself more, challenging yourself more with your daily cardio and fitness routine.

9. *Weigh yourself every dang day.* Period. No compromises on this one. It's like daily walking, breathing, and brushing your teeth. You get my drift. Use that number on the scale to motivate yourself to remind yourself where you came from and where you want to be for the rest of your life.

Chapter 22

Ideas to Keep You on Track

"Perseverance is not a long race; it is many short races - one after another."

—*Walter Elliott, American Catholic priest and author*

Every day is like a race for me: a quest for perseverance, for excellence with my diet, daily cardio, and everything else I'm involved in. Take new diet and fitness plans, for instance. In preparation for making sure I persevere and stick to mine throughout the year, I just flushed what was left of a bag of sugar-free chocolate covered bridge mix down my garbage disposal.

Why? Because I can't stand the thought of the power that kind of stuff sometimes has over me, and I'm not taking any chances. The fact that they're sugar free means nothing to my pancreas. Seems it's so used to existing on white starches and sugar from my old, fat days that the slightest bit of sugar-free chemical trickery sends it into overdrive once again.

I don't wait until next Monday or Tuesday or any other day to wean myself off those deadly carbs; I start right away. Who else in their right mind would flush chocolate-covered nuts down the garbage disposal?

Don't wait till next week to make your new health and fitness plans; get on them now. Write them down and reread them every single day, until you get it. Stop mucking around and get that unhealthy, unwanted weight off once and for all. You know you can do it and I'm here to help you.

Begin by asking yourself, "What have I accomplished so far this year, health- and fitness-wise?" And if you're not satisfied with your answer, and if you're staring at rising insurance costs due to your weight, try some of the many tips I've given you in this book.

Thirty Seconds to Thirty Minutes a Day

Sometimes it's easier to break tasks into short, doable chunks. You can look at your health and fitness program in the same way. Just look at the positive, healthy, and fun activities you can perform in short blocks of time.

30 seconds

- The time it takes to make a healthier food choice than you normally would. Put that bagel back on the rack and reach for an apple and a piece of cheese to hold hunger at bay between meals. Keep it low white starch and sugar carb.

- The time it takes to slip the top and bottom buns from your lusciously juicy burger or the two pieces of bread surrounding that deli sandwich. You don't need the extra carbs (no matter what the Subway guy says, who seemed to regain much of his weight until his sponsors got him running to lose it again). It's the white starch and sugar in the bread, buns, chips and desserts that's killing you, kids! Duh. Have a light, sugar-free, carb-free dessert instead. Strawberries and real cream, anyone?

30 – 60 seconds

- The time it takes to call your waitress/waiter back because your conscience got the better of you and now you want to change your order to something more low-carb, low-fat, and health conscious than fried chicken and mashed potatoes. Good going! Your body and pancreas will love you for it.

- The time it takes to talk yourself into putting that half gallon of ice cream back in the freezer—before you heap it in a bowl and gobble it down or snarf it right from the cold carton—before you even know what hit you.

- Weigh yourself every single morning, then let those numbers sink into your mind as you record them in your health and fitness journal. I really can't stress the importance of this enough.

60 seconds to 5 minutes

- The time it could take to talk a friend into walking with you.

60 seconds to 30 minutes

- The time it takes to buy your new pair of walking shoes—the best pair you can afford.

2 minutes

- The time it takes to lace up your brand new walking shoes, strap on your fanny pack, and get out the door for your walk.

1 to 3 minutes

- Get up and go get it yourself, whatever it is. No matter if it's a piece of paper you need from a co-worker sitting a short distance away (or a floor away), a cup of coffee, something copied or faxed, or a treat from the store—get up and move. Get it for yourself. Do it for the health of it. And it better be low carb!

3 minutes

- The time it takes to whip yourself up a low-carb, high-protein shake to stave off hunger's temptation and satisfy that sweet snacking urge. Especially mid-afternoon.

5 minutes

- The time it takes to nuke a low-carb frozen entrée when you need a bit of help with low-cal, low-carb portion control. It's a no brainer. No seconds or thirds, here. What you see is what you eat.

10 minutes

- The time it takes to make a great big fresh salad instead of having a bowl of cereal or a buttered bagel for a solo dinner or midnight snack. Nocturnal noshing not allowed!

10 to 30 minutes a day

- Take your dog/dogs for a nice, well-deserved walk. They will love you for it. If you don't have a dog, borrow one!

- Take a lunchtime walk, a morning walk, an extra walk, or walk to and from the train, bus, or car.

- Time spent writing in your fitness journal affirming your health, diet, fitness, and special life goals.

- Religiously practice your Pilates, yoga, or various home-exercise routines on the days you don't go to the health club. Do whatever it takes to improve your stability and flexibility and get your heart rate up. Better yet, take a walk. There's nothing like daily cardio.

20 to 30 minutes

- Performing weight training a minimum of three times a week works wonders for your well-being, strength, fitness, and stamina.

- The optimum time it takes to practice daily meditation for increased willpower, courage, clarity, creativity, stamina, and help with anything and everything in your life.

30 minutes (realistically 60 minutes) a day

- The time it takes for daily walking to make you feel better and look even younger and more gorgeous than you've ever dreamed possible, and keep you that way for as long as you continue to walk and stick to a healthy diet.

Chapter 23

Ask Laura

"A person who never made a mistake never tried anything new."

—*Albert Einstein*
German-born physicist and pillar of modern physics

Dear Laura:

I fell off my diet and fitness wagon and I'm back at 159 lbs.! I started following your advice about a year ago when I was at 162 lbs. and went down to 139 lbs., but now I'm up again. I never really allowed myself to reach my goal of 125-130, which would be wonderful for my petite height. I think my hormones are playing a big part. I started premenopause. (Keep it a secret, it makes me feel like I'm entering middle age).

I had lost my weight and maintained it on *The South Beach Diet*, but didn't stick to it all during the week, like you advise. I failed to make it my lifestyle. Do you think I should go back to that diet? I need your words of motivation and advice.

—D

Dear D:

If you're lookin' for the "Easy Button" of diet, health, and fitness plans, there ain't one. My biggest words of advice: get back on that low-carb diet ASAP. Cut the dang white starch and sugar carbs; you know this by now. And squeeze in that hour of cardio every single day, no matter what the "experts" say. A good, healthy, effective diet/lifestyle eating plan and daily cardio go hand in hand. Period. Anything less than an hour a day and you're just spinning your wheels. You know what works for you from your last dieting attempt with *The South Beach Diet*. Low-carb. You had tremendous success with it. Why not try it again? Or go Atkins, my ultimate favorite.

Get your SB diet book out and reread the quick start and begin again, right now, for your very next meal. Either you're gonna do it, or you're not. You forgot that what worked for you in the first place was cutting the carbs. Carbs are your enemy, *not* dietary fat. Insulin's the "fat hormone." Do some serious soul searching to see where you're going wrong with your eating, and no fair blaming it on hormones. Don't get me started there. It's your carb consumption, girlfriend, pure and simple.

~ ~ ~

Hi Laura:

I came across your article in an old edition of *First for Women* magazine and immediately went to your website.

I am fifty-seven years old, 5'6", and would like to lose twenty-five pounds. I started walking two and a half weeks ago and walk three to four mph for about forty-five minutes every day. My question is: when typically do the pounds start to come off? Most of my extra weight is in my abdomen.

I appreciate any of your knowledge and help.

Thank you.

—MC

Dear MC:

Thank your shiny stars that twenty-five pounds is all you need to lose, you lucky stiff. I know many who live for the day when they'll be able to slip into your slimmer shoes.

Two and a half weeks of walking isn't nearly enough time for your body to get the message that you're trying to turn it into a highly efficient, fat-burning machine.

If you're walking every day and maintaining the speed and intensity that you say you are during the entire forty-five minutes, you should see some results in no time. But you need a little patience and a little more time. And you cannot exercise away a bad diet; if you're not following a good, sensible, healthy, effective eating plan along with your daily walking regimen, you could hike from here to the Hamptons and you'd just be spinning your wheels—you won't lose an ounce.

So, if I were you, I'd bump those forty-five minutes up to an hour a day as soon as you can. When you want to boil weight off, it takes real effort. If you can do three to four miles a day to begin with, you're just getting fired up. Five miles a day is optimum, and if you can do more in a second walk that day, it's even better.

Another benefit is that the more you walk, the less crap you'll want to eat. Cravings for a lot of the stuff that keep you fat start to disappear. But you do have to combine your daily walking with a good, effective, healthy diet—preferably low carb. (I sound like a broken CD here!)

What "beginning walking" is for you—starting with forty-five minutes at fifteen- to twenty-minute miles—is not "beginning walking" to a person just starting out who has fifty or 100-plus pounds to lose. Maybe some haven't moved any further than the fridge in eons so they'll be lucky to get in ten to fifteen minutes at a time, but that's okay. You gotta start somewhere.

What matters most for each one of us, however, no matter how much weight we have to lose, no matter what kind of shape we're in, is that we begin to make walking a daily habit right now and keep going for as long as we can move.

Have a big belly? Got double chins? How about an ass and thighs that could eclipse the sun, if given the chance? No problemo. Daily walking mysteriously ferrets out all the visceral fat—that goopy, glucky, nasty stuff that lurks, surrounds, and chokes off our vital organs—and just magically melts it away. You won't believe how your body will miraculously change once you begin to walk daily.

But it does take time. You didn't pack on the pounds overnight, so they're not coming off overnight, either. If you stick with this whole daily walking and diet thing like I advise, if you are completely honest with yourself and give it a chance, suddenly you'll begin to hear comments from your friends and others like, "Wow, what're you doing with yourself these days? You look awesome! Betcha feel great!"

And you'll smile when you hear yourself say with a wink, "C'mon, girlie, take a walk with me and I'll tell ya all about it."

~ ~ ~

The following is a portion of a wonderful letter I received from one of my readers (T).

T: Dear Laura: I would like to share my story with you and your readers. I woke up one morning in January and I was tired of being fat and tired all the time.

Laura: This is exactly what it takes to get started on your health and fitness transformation. It has to come from inside of you. You have to become fed up with your life the way it is. You have to be ready for change.

T: I decided to watch what I ate (no more junk food) and knew I needed to come up with an exercise plan.

Laura: It's great that you realize diet alone will not help you shed the pounds that you want and keep them off.

T: Plus, I drink a lot of water (just one diet soda on the weekend).

Laura: I cannot stress the importance of drinking enough water throughout your day. It keeps you hydrated so that everything on the inside works at its optimum, keeps your joints "oiled," gets rid of all the waste, and my personal favorite: plumps the skin on your face like nothing else. A good friend of mine, a longtime Weight Watchers devotee, insists that the people who consistently lose the most weight at the weekly weigh-ins are the ones who drink the most water.

T: I started out walking every day after work with one mile. I increased it by a half of a mile by the end of the first week. Each week I added another half a mile. I am now walking six miles a day. On the weekdays, I do a minimum of three miles outside and three miles on the treadmill.

Laura: Your walking accomplishment is stellar and I'm glad that I helped motivate you to make the commitment to make daily walking a part of your total health and fitness plan. Increasing your walking distance by adding a half-mile a week is quite a big enchilada. You discovered you could handle it and were comfortable doing so without hurting yourself. Bravo.

Everyone has different limitations. Each has to find her/his own place, then work past it to achieve optimum fat-burning results. Walking every day becomes such an ingrained healthy habit that, if you're tempted to blow it off when your life gets in the way, you won't be able to. You know how well daily walking serves you.

T: I have a disabled child and work at a school for disabled children. At the time I decided to lose weight, they had a contest at work for the biggest loser. The first place loser would win a trip to Key West and the second-place loser would win the cash that everyone put in the pot ($10 each = $280 total). I was the first place winner. In twelve weeks I lost thirty-seven pounds and four dress sizes. Since then I have lost six more pounds.

Laura: What an enormous achievement. Congratulations! I know you're going to enjoy yourself in Margaritaville. Have one for all of us!

T: Walking is physical and mental therapy for me.

Laura: To say that walking is physical and mental therapy is an understatement. The benefits of daily walking far outweigh almost every other form of exercise. I know firsthand; I've tried it all.

T: I am having some problems about still feeling fat, though. I have to keep looking at myself in the mirror to remind me that I am small. I have been fat for twenty-five years. I have a picture of myself on the refrigerator and in the living room to help keep me motivated.

Laura: Do what you have to do, my dear friend, to reassure yourself that you are one of the most beautiful gals around. You are gorgeous, healthy, and fabulously fit, inside now as well as out.

And, sadly, sometimes we still see ourselves with "fat eyes" no matter how much weight we lose. It's just one of those things, but you have to learn to know in your heart that you're fat no more—and eat and act accordingly.

As you walk and get into your meditative state, tell yourself, "I am the best. I deserve the best. I am strong, healthy, vibrant, and more beautiful than ever." Say this over and over and over. Then believe it.

It definitely takes a while for your mind to catch up with your body. I still have days when I feel fat. It's a hard demon to shake. Mine's been with me since early childhood. Keep looking in the mirror. Say it to the mirror. Believe what you see.

T: I live in hurricane alley and I was wondering how I could stay on a low-fat diet when eating canned food because of no electricity? Depending on how bad our town is hit, walking might be a problem, too.

Laura: If I were you, I'd stock up on low-carb, low-glycemic veggie staples like canned green beans, spinach, etc. Water-packed tuna in the can or pouch, apples, almonds and other nuts should be high on your list, also. Forget the chips and pokey-bait snack foods, and I mean it. There are a lot of other things you can come up with to eat that aren't carb-laden, empty calories.

Stash as much bottled water as you can lay your hands on. And I'm sure you'll find a safe way to walk after the storm's fury passes. I know I'd be out there as soon as I possibly could.

T: I am very happy with my progress, and I do not want to go back to the way I was.

Laura: I don't blame you. Sustaining your weight loss can be one of the most difficult things you've ever done. Or it doesn't have to be. It's strictly up to you. Every time you're tempted to eat carby crap, ask yourself: how badly do I want to maintain my new, healthier weight?

You know exactly what it took to get the pounds off; now modify that and do what it takes to keep them off. Stick to your healthy eating plan during the week and learn to be satisfied with one normal helping of your favorite foods on the weekend—dinners only, not three belt-busters a day. The pounds you'll pack back on by Monday won't be worth it.

T: I enjoyed your article in *First for Women* as well as the motivational blog articles that you write. I share them all with my coworkers. My friends at work were afraid that I was not eating because I dropped the weight real fast. But I eat and I am eating healthy. My family is now watching what they eat and getting on the treadmill, too.

Laura: If you ate a healthy balanced diet that was low in white starchy, sugary carbs and fat, and included the amount of daily walking you say you did, it's no wonder your weight fell off. Invite your co-workers to join you for lunchtime walks so they can experience the benefits of daily walking firsthand. Then start a daily walking club.

It's also wonderful that your family is following in your healthy footsteps. Positive role models should always begin at home. There's nothing more powerful than setting a good example for your family and friends. I wish more people would take the bull by the horns like you and I did and stop making excuses for why they're fat. Changing their eating and exercise habits would drastically improve their lives.

T: Thank you for all your motivational articles and such, and keep on walking.

Best regards, T

Laura: Thank you, T, for your encouragement. All the best on your health and fitness quest.

~ ~ ~

On a Saturday evening not too long ago, we were at a party where I met the woman (Ann), who wrote the following letter to me the next day. She sat a few seats away from me at our table. Her letter demonstrates the level of motivational enthusiasm I am able to inspire in others.

Ann: Hi Laura, My name is Ann. I met you at the party last night; we were sitting at the same table. I just wanted to thank you again for your *Commit To Get Fit* book. I've read most of it already and really enjoy it. I hope to finish reading it by this evening. I also spent some time reading the articles on your website and blog today. Somewhere between the two places, I read that it takes five weeks to make a healthy diet and fitness a habit. Well Laura, today is day one!

Laura: Congratulations, girl! This is exactly what it takes: one day at a time determination and walking, even in the rain, so grab an umbrella. Because of my daily walking, I have come to love the outdoors and all its glorious weather even more than ever. As long as you can walk, you can go anywhere.

Ann: As soon as I send you this e-mail, I've got my walking shoes on and I'm off to walk around a lake by our house.

Laura: Great! The real key here is to do it; walk every single day, no matter what. And do as much as you can each day. If you can't walk first thing in the morning, grab some steps at lunch or squeeze some in after dinner. You already know all the standard tried-and-true tricks to wedge walking in where you can. Park far away. Take the stairs. Blah. Blah. Blah. But, you have to carve out <u>real</u> walking time for yourself and make it fit <u>your</u> schedule. I know you're a mom; I know you're a wife. I also know you're a "You." And now that "You" needs to be taken care of. Make the time every single day.

Don't hurt yourself by doing too much all at once. Gently build up distance and time every week. Learn to compete with *yourself.* No one else matters. Remember: it's not a race - it's a parade. And please get a digital step counter (pedometer) of some sort. For options, please see the resources pages at the back of this book. I've been known to wear my step counter everywhere, still, and keep a daily record, to this day—just because I can. I love to track my progress and I need the inspiration and motivation. I logged nine miles the other day. If you don't think that motivates me when I see that number in my fitness journal, think again.

I have so much to tell you and others in this book about how to continue walking and make it a lifelong habit, how to keep on target even when things gets tough, how to see this through to the end, and how to maintain it. And BTW, I'm in my tenth year of maintenance. Please feel free to e-mail me when you need a quick kick in the butt, have questions, or whatever. I am always here for you.

Ann: I'm really glad I got to talk to you about this last night.

Laura: And so am I. As soon as I laid eyes on you, I knew you were ready. You will set a great example for your husband, too. He could use a bit of reduction around his "Equator."

Ann: I just have to do this whether I have my head together or not ...

Laura: Daily walking will help you get your head together. Learn to meditate. I have lots of resources for you in the back of this book and on my website. Ideally, one should meditate first thing in the morning. And, yes, before your walk. Lots to cram into a day, but your life will vastly improve. Think about all the time-wasting, unproductive things you do in a day and use that time to walk. Once you get it down to a routine, you'll feel like you're flying by the time you finish. And, your head will come together faster. Everything will be easier.

Ann: I'm so tired of being overweight . .

Laura: Isn't that the truth? So was I. I was simply tired of hauling myself around.

Ann: I figure I can do anything for thirty-five straight days. And by then it should be something I feel I want to do . .

Laura: You seriously can do this. Thirty-five days is a piece of cake, especially when you begin to see results. Let nothing stand in your way, not even Sunday mornings. Get out and do it, just because you can. And it's not easy every day. Some days I have one heck of a time getting out that door for my walk. But before you know it, you're into it, and after you finish, you'll be so glad you did it and didn't blow it off that I can't even begin to tell you.

I have a wonderful, six- and twelve-week private or group support program available. In it I cover meditation, walking, the right diet for you, and everything else you'll need to make this time your last time. You know what I mean. I certainly don't have all the answers, but I do know what has worked and NOT worked for me for over fifty years and now I can share all the knowledge and information I've gained with you.

You are so beautiful and lovely. I know you're doing this for yourself, but your family will also benefit from your increased health and fitness long term.

Ann: Thanks and have a great week!

Laura: You, too! And remember, today is Day 2. The next day is Day 3 and, before you even know it, it'll be your thirty-fifth day. Then you've got it made—if you want to. It's all up to you.

Appendices

The Low-Carb Lifestyle

The two main types of harmful carbohydrates are sugars and starches—all the white stuff. In order to lose weight the low-carb way, keep your carbohydrate count for the day to around thirty to thirty-five grams. It isn't a lot of carbs, but it is a lot of food.

At the very beginning of my diet, since I had such a tremendous amount of weight to lose and I was literally living a lifetime on high-carb, low-fat foods, I did not count the carbs in whole milk (which I personally prefer because of my finicky stomach and for my skin). I also didn't count the carbs in tomatoes because if I was going to now include a big salad every day in my diet, I'd count my carb allotment for the day in all the white starch and sugar foods I was previously eating that kept me fat and were slowly killing me. This was just enough to get me into successful weight-loss mode.

I figured that was sacrifice enough for me to really get myself started and it proved a wise decision on my part. Once I began to see real results—it didn't happen overnight, but it didn't take all that long, either—I became even more motivated.

My weight-loss journey was like that proverbial little snowball rolling down the hill. The further it went, the bigger it got, gaining momentum all the while, until pretty soon—success! And, before you know it, you'll be into your own weight-loss success story, too.

Study the following foods listed and avoid them at all costs. They truly are what is keeping you fat.

Eat more protein and low-glycemic fruits and veggies, drink lots of water, and exercise daily. Develop these healthy habits for life. And, as with any health and fitness plan, please be sure to consult with your doctor before you begin. And take your Flintstone's chewable or Gummy multivitamins every day. I do. Some days I chew two.

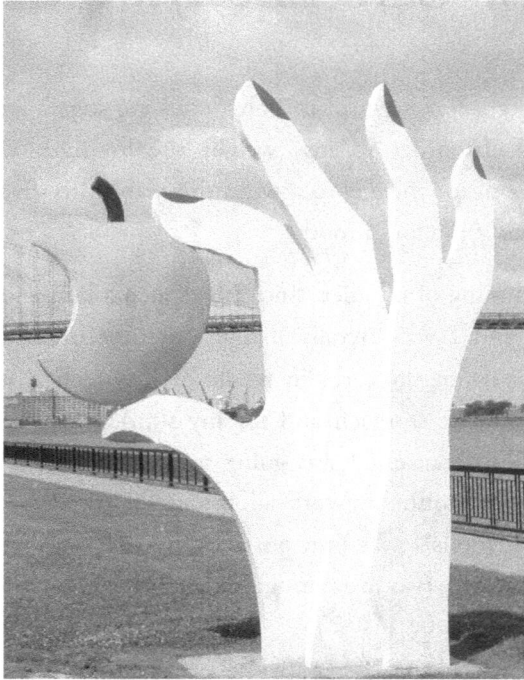

Eat an apple a day for the health of it.
(Sculpture credit: Eve's Apple by Edwina Sandys,
One of Two: Gift to the city of Windsor, Ontario, Canada)

Foods to Avoid Like the Plague

All bread—including whole wheat, rolls, sweet rolls, hot dog and hamburger buns, pizza crust, pasta, macaroni & cheese, ravioli, grits, white rice, brown rice, Spanish rice, tortillas, tamales, chips, taco chips, nacho chips, potato chips, popcorn, all snack foods, French fries, curly fries, onion rings. Get the picture?

Avoid *all* breaded and deep-fried foods; pull the breading off of everything. It won't kill you. Otherwise, you'll be wearing it

Avoid potatoes, white and sweet, mashed, fried, boiled, candied, yams, sweet potato pie, all pies, cakes, cookies, pancakes, waffles, candies. Cereals of all kinds—especially oatmeal, Cheerios, Special K, and granola—are not on this diet.

Avoid diet cheese, cheese spreads, or whey cheeses. People with a yeast infection, dairy allergy, or lactose intolerance must avoid cheese. Imitation cheese products are not allowed, except for tofu (soy cheese), but always check carbohydrate content.

Avoid energy and power bars that are not low-carb. Ethnic foods that contain white starch and sugar, such as empanadas, enchiladas, etc., and anything from Taco Bell and the like are mostly high-carb poison. They cause your pancreas to overproduce insulin—the fat hormone. It's not the fat in food that makes you fat, it's the white starch and sugar carbs.

Also avoid ice creams, milk shakes, and yogurt sweetened with fruit (eat only plain Greek yogurt or whole-milk yogurt). You'll get used to it and then crave the tartness of it, trust me on this one. Add your own fresh fruit so you can control the carbs. Stay away from syrups, jellies and jams, soda pop, Coke, Pepsi, Mountain Dew (don't), and chocolate milk. Sorry. You'll soon get over it. Alcoholic beverages are not part of the beginning induction phase of the diet.

Avoid high-glycemic fruits and veggies, such as corn, potatoes, peas, carrots, bananas, oranges, watermelon, pineapple, grapes, most beans at first (until you lose your weight), refried beans, etc. Do not drink fruit juices, *or* at least cut all juices in half with club soda if you absolutely have to drink them; they're all loaded with sugar. If it's high glycemic or high carb, avoid it all. Seriously.

Artificial Sweeteners

Dieters must determine which artificial sweeteners agree with them. Eventually you will lose your taste for anything artificially sweetened, and it is my hope for you that you can get used to the taste of a natural, no-carb alternative called Stevia and a natural sweetening product called Truvia (available in most supermarkets). It's made from the leaf of a tree grown in South America. I use it in liquid form every day in my coffee, tea, and lemonade that I make with organic Italian Lemon Juice from Costco. You have to play with the proportions until you get them right for your taste buds, so pay attention if you use it. A little can go a long, long way.

Use no natural sweeteners ending in the letters "ose," such as maltose and fructose. Fructose, as in high-fructose corn syrup, is especially deadly to a low-carb lifestyle. Talk about fueling an addiction.

Aspartame, found in Nutra-Sweet and Equal, requires a special note of explanation. Whereas virtually all published scientific studies (many sponsored by the drug companies that make them) show aspartame to be safe, there has been a great volume of word-of-mouth complaints attesting to its potential risks: headaches, irritability, seizure disorder, and vision problems, among others, have all been claimed.

Dr. Atkin's concern about aspartame is its possible adverse effect on sugar metabolism and weight. He took scores of aspartame users, who appeared metabolically resistant to weight loss, off this sweetener and observed weight loss resume. As a result of the studies, he recommends its use in small quantities (less than three packets of Equal or equivalent daily). People with known sensitivity to MSG should avoid it at all costs. Personally, I avoid it all like poison.

Also, from my own personal experience: all those artificial sweeteners are deadly. They're neurotoxins (brain poison). Google them and read about them if you're concerned about your overall health and well-being. And you should be. Otherwise, why bother?

I never counted a calorie or fat gram to lose my 130 pounds in two and a half years. Ever. I only counted the carbohydrate content in each food that I ate and subtracted the fiber for my total carb count. And look what a modified Atkins Diet did, and continues to do, for me to this day.

A calorie may be a calorie, but when you're carb sensitive, if a food is low in calories but high in carbs, stay away from it. Those low-calorie, low-fat, high-carb foods will surely pack on the pounds when you're trying to shave them off. Would I lie to you? And stay away from anything super-sized. Why do you need a super or large size of anything, when a small or medium size will satisfy your hunger, taste, thirst, and dietary food budget?

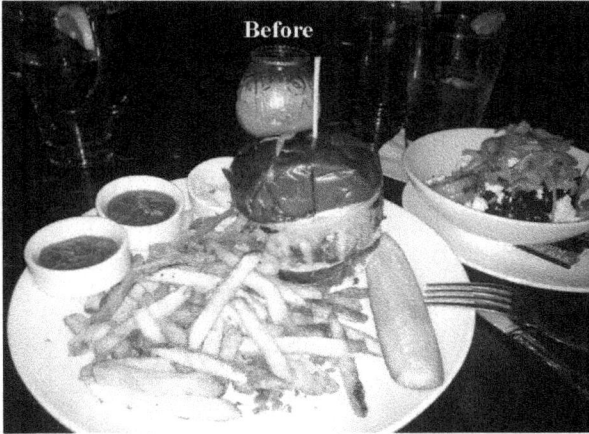

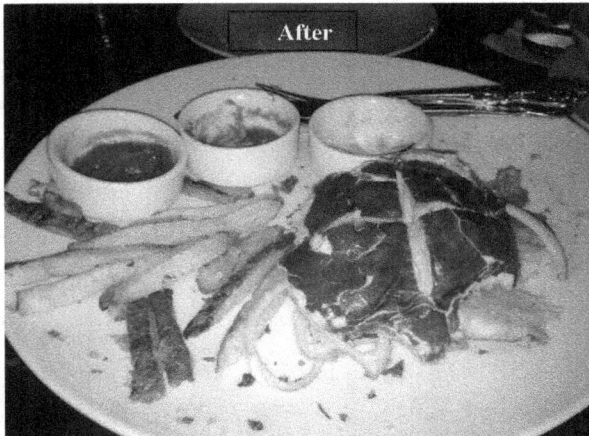

Remember your new mantra: "Eat the burger, not the bun, eat the sandwich innards, not all the bread or roll, eat the cheese, sausage and everything else off the top of the pizza, but never, ever eat the bottom crust."

As with any new diet, health and fitness plan, please be sure to consult with your doctor before you begin.

Common Mistakes to Avoid

Note that the 14-day Atkins Diet that I followed at the time contains no fruit. However, per my doctor's request, I ate two servings a day of low-glycemic fruits: apples, strawberries, cantaloupe, and honeydew melon. I had the melons at breakfast time and the apple later in the afternoon with cheese and almonds, or strawberries with plain, whole-milk yogurt sweetened with liquid Stevia, for a great snack. The 14-day diet also contains no bread, grains, starchy vegetables, or dairy products, other than cottage cheese, cheese, cream or butter. Note: I added whole milk and cottage cheese because I had to. Otherwise, I also ate low fat as much as I could.

Avoid diet products unless they specifically state "No carbohydrates." Most dietetic foods are for fat-restricted, not carbohydrate-restricted, diets. Just because a food is labeled low fat doesn't mean it's low-carb. Beware. Read the carb content—always—on everything. The word "sugarless" is not sufficient. The product must state the carbohydrate content, and that's what you go by. Many products you do not normally think of as food, such as chewing gum, cough syrups, and cough drops, are filled with sugar or other caloric sweeteners and must be avoided.

Now, what you really need to do is go out and buy your own copy of the *The NEW Atkins For A New You, The ULTIMATE DIET for SHEDDING WEIGHT and FEELING GREAT* (see the Resources section), so that you can see all this information in its proper context as it was written and how it's intended to be used—as a roadmap to better health and well-being and a total lifestyle for the rest of your life.

Low-Carb Food List

To count your carbs accurately, a comprehensive carbohydrate and fat gram counting guide like *The Diabetes Carbohydrate and Fat Gram Guide* by Lea Ann Holzmeister, RD, CDE, is a handy reference guide. Atkins has an excellent one, as well. I highlight all my favorite foods and refer to both books often. The following is a list of good-for-you foods to help you kick your carbohydrate addiction (and habit).

Beverages: water, spring water, mineral water, club soda, essence flavored seltzer (must say "no calories"), decaffeinated coffee or tea, clear broth/bouillon (not all brands), and cream (heavy or light, just note carbohydrate content). Caffeine mimics the effect of sugar on blood glucose levels by stimulating insulin release. It should be avoided by those who suspect they are caffeine dependent and taken in limited quantities by others. And I'm guilty here because my beverage of choice is a café latte—and I have two 20- oz. half-caf lattes with 2% milk each day. This is one of my only vices. Could be worse. Choose yours wisely.

Eggs - Chicken, goose, quail, ostrich, and duck.

Dairy - All cheeses have some carbohydrate content, and quantities are governed by that. My personal favorites are Manchego (a yummy sheep-milk gouda from Spain), Italian Friulano, fontina, bleu, gorgonzola, Swiss, goat, cheddar, you name it. As far as cheeses go, I probably like it—a lot! Cream cheese is also a given. Unsweetened whipped cream and whole milk are acceptable in limited quantities.

Fish – Trout, salmon, halibut, haddock, smelt, herring, mackerel, sardines, and perch.

Fruits – Cantaloupe, honeydew melon, strawberries, blueberries, raspberries, black raspberries, rhubarb, avocado, apricot, currants, guava, olives, and prunes (but *no* fruit juices).

Herbs – Thyme, rosemary, oregano, basil, cilantro, and marjoram.

Lean meat – Grass-fed beef, elk, buffalo, goat, pork, lamb, deer, moose, and jerky.

Nuts/seeds – Pecans, almonds, cashews, walnuts, pistachios, macadamia, and hazelnuts, as well as pumpkin and sunflower seeds.

Oils – Olive, flaxseed, avocado, coconut, and walnut.

Poultry – Chicken (skinless), turkey, duck, pheasant, quail, and ostrich.

Seafood – Shrimp, crab, lobster, scallops, clams, squid, eel, octopus, and mussels. And you know those "fake crab sticks?" Well, it turns out that they're made from haddock, one of the *best* fish you could ever eat. So, don't hesitate to go faux!

Vegetables – Artichokes, green beans, broccoli, celery, asparagus, cabbage, chard, kale, spinach, lettuce, Brussels sprouts (try them roasted!), rhubarb, squash, onions, cucumbers, peppers, eggplant, zucchini, leeks, tomatoes, and cauliflower.

Low-Carb Meal Suggestions

Your aim for eating is to strive for low-calorie, high-density foods. By this, I mean you want to eat foods that are low in carbohydrates but take up a lot of space. These types of food have a low-caloric value due, in part, to the lower amount of carbohydrates in them, but they take up a larger volume of space than other foods do. For example, you can eat a small order of French fries at your favorite fast-food place and it will have about 275 calories and thirty grams of carbohydrates. However, they will not come close to filling you up and holding off your hunger pains for very long. Or, you can eat a medium-size salad with fresh greens, vegetables, and maybe some protein in the form of meat or fish. That salad will contain approximately the same calories as those French fries but fewer than five grams of carbohydrates and it will keep you full for hours.

It's really quite simple, if you think about it. Some other examples would be one chocolate chip cookie or all the sugar-free Jell-O you can possibly eat. You could eat a four-ounce bowl of corn flakes, which is about 400 calories and also has over 100 grams of carbohydrates in it. Or, you could eat five eggs for the same 400 calories yet only consume about three grams of carbohydrates. Maybe you like lasagna? A decent serving of lasagna has almost 700 calories and seventy grams of carbohydrates, but for those same 700 calories you could eat about fourteen ounces of grilled or baked salmon and consume zero carbohydrates. Get the picture?

Breakfast

- Eggs – Omelets, scrambled, fried, frittata, crustless quiche, or poached. Mix in some ham and/or veggies. Add some bacon or turkey sausage. Just forget about the toast—even whole wheat.

- Greek yogurt, cottage cheese, cream cheese, ricotta, or tofu. Sweeten with Stevia and add low-glycemic fruit to it, if you like.

- Protein shakes – Whatever flavor you like, but make sure it's low carb. Many are not. Smoothies and protein shakes are trigger foods for me, so I try to stay totally away from them. All I wanna do after I finish one is have another one—and I like to chew, so I'm then looking for something to gnaw on to satisfy that chomping craving.

- Meat – Nothing wrong with having a burger (without the bun of course), ham, sausage, turkey burger, or steak for breakfast to get some protein in your system.

- Fish – Salmon, white fish, tuna, or shrimp are a great way to start the day. You have to unwrap your mind from what you know to be the "traditional" breakfast meal. Customize the low-carb diet to suit you.

Lunch

- Hamburgers/cheeseburgers/poultry – Just don't eat the bun. Give the bun to the birds.

- Soups – There are lots of low-carb soups available; just read the labels and get those that are low in carbohydrates and sodium.

- Salads – Fresh greens with some sliced grilled chicken, ham, or steak. Leave off the salad dressing that contains carbs. Low-calorie ranch, Thousand Island, and even French are not the answer. Low calorie doesn't mean low carb. For salad dressing, I use my desired oil plus vinegar or lemon juice and spices. Grated cheese, bleu cheese, chopped eggs, bacon, or sour cream may be added.

- Leftovers – Your leftovers from your low-carb dinner the night before will always work the next day for breakfast or lunch. You'll be surprised how long into the day your breakfast of leftover Chilean sea bass and sautéed broccoli will hold you.

- Tuna/Salmon/Egg Salad – Make sandwiches with Romaine lettuce leaves instead of bread. "Unwich" those sandwiches and lose the breads and tortilla-type wraps. (There goes your thirty to thirty-five grams of carbs for the day. It's so not worth it, if you ask me.) Get creative and add in some of your favorite spices or herbs to amp up the taste. Just fill a leaf with the salad mix and eat it like you're eating a hot dog.

Dinner

- Meat – Chicken, turkey, beef, lamb, and pork. There are hundreds of ways to prepare your favorite types and cuts of meat. Marinate it or add some herbs and spices for seasoning. Grill it, bake it, roast it, or fry it. Add in some veggies for a delicious low-carb dinner the whole family will enjoy.

- Fish – Salmon, tuna, white-meat types of fish, shrimp, crab, and lobster can all be prepared and cooked just like the meats already mentioned.

- Dinner salads – Get creative and make a large dinner salad with fresh greens, low-carb veggies, and sliced chicken, beef, turkey, fish, or pork. Add some sliced hard-boiled eggs and your favorite low-carb salad dressing and you're good to go.

- Casseroles – Everything mentioned in this section can be made into a delicious casserole. The variations and ingredients are endless. Put on your thinking cap and come up with some casseroles you and your family would love. Do you need some suggestions or help with preparing your casserole? Checkout the following link for some great casserole recipes: www.yummly.com/recipes/low-carb-casseroles.

- Eating out at restaurants – Most restaurant chains and independent restaurants now list or have special sections for their low-carb meal offerings. The following link will help you find which restaurant chains have low-carb fare: lowcarbdiets.about.com/od/eatingout/.

Desserts

- Low-carb brownie mixes – there are now several companies that sell a low-carb brownie mixes that taste as good as the normal high-carb versions—like Atkins!

- Sugar-free Jell-O – Mix it with whipped cream or cottage cheese or have it by itself.

- Chocolate – Has to be above 70% cocoa. (After all, isn't chocolate in its own food group?)

- Low-carb cheesecake – Low-carb mixes for this delicious dessert are available and The Cheesecake Factory has low-carb cheesecake on their menu. If you're eating there, you can order a low-carb dinner, too.

- Search the Internet – There a hundreds and hundreds of recipes on the Internet for many types of low-carb dessert recipes that include cakes, pies, puddings, mousses, custards, and cheesecakes.

Snacks

- Celery w/peanut butter – Cut some celery into four-inch-long pieces and fill with a couple of tablespoons of peanut butter. (Tip: Trader Joe's has one of the best tasting, low-carb versions around: Valencia Peanuts with Roasted Flax Seeds.)

- Nuts – A quarter cup of unsalted nuts or mixed nuts is a nice snack once or twice a day.

- Sugar-free Jell-O – Mix your favorite flavor with some whipped cream, cottage cheese, or just by itself.

- Jerky – Either beef or turkey. Try to find brands with minimal sugar.

- Rollups – Wrap a slice of turkey breast around a piece of celery or mozzarella cheese stick. You can also use prosciutto, salami, or lean roast beef.

- Veggies – Cucumbers, lettuce, celery, mushrooms, green/red/yellow peppers, cauliflower, and broccoli. Stay away from carrots; they're too high glycemic. Try having your veggies with a little whipped cream cheese if you want. Want to have or serve a tasty low-carb dip with your veggies? Try some of the low-carb dips from the following link: www.yummly.com/recipes/low-carb-vegetable-dip

Appetizers

Here are some ideas for delicious low-carb appetizers to create and experiment with. Since everyone's tastes vary, you can do an Internet search to get different recipe ideas and ingredients to try for each one of these.

Artichoke Dip

Prosciutto Wrapped Asparagus

Marinated Grilled Shrimp

Hummus Dip

Salsa

Guacamole

Chicken Enchilada Dip

Jalapeno Poppers

Ham or Salami Cream Cheese Rollups

Parmesan or Mozzarella Broccoli Balls

Lobster Dip

Meatballs

Stuffed Mushrooms

Spinach Brownies

Fresh Veggies

Pizza Dip

Deviled Eggs

Spinach Dip

Cheese Ball with Nuts

Sausage Cheese Balls

Vegetarian Low-Carb Recipe Ideas

Contributed by Lisa Eby, Elgin, IL

Yes, it is possible to eat low-carb vegetarian and still lose weight. Get creative. Just cut the carbs. Some vegetarians are concerned that they may not be able to live a satisfying low-carb lifestyle. By using some important substitutions, nearly any recipe can be turned into a low-carb vegetarian one. The following recipes will give you some ideas about altered favorites that will still allow you to lose weight.

Grilled Portabellas

Marinate large portabella mushrooms in a bit of olive oil plus three to four times more balsamic vinegar mixed with Italian spices (or just use balsamic salad dressing in bottle). Grill or broil portabellas until almost done, then sprinkle inside of cap with thawed soy sausage crumbles and/or shredded Parmesan, bleu, or feta cheese. Broil until cheese melts. Serve with salad and/or fresh, steamed green veggies.

Alternate: Skip the veggie crumbles and go for a veggie burger instead. Sprinkle the veggie burger with Parmesan, bleu, or feta cheese and top with grilled/broiled portabella. Dip each bite in a bit of stone-ground mustard for an additional taste treat.

If you like a variety of tastes in a meal, splurge with just a bit of poppy seed salad dressing—since you were careful with the rest of your meal, treat yourself.

Veggie Lasagna

Preheat oven to 375°F.

Wipe 9"x13" glass baking dish with thin coat olive oil.

Layer:

- Tomato sauce mixed with Italian seasoning to taste.

- Sliced zucchini (slice lengthwise to simulate lasagna noodles)

- Diced fresh or canned tomatoes

- Soy sausage crumbles (whole package)

- Repeat tomato sauce mixture

- Grated Parmesan cheese

- Repeat sliced zucchini

- Repeat diced fresh or canned tomatoes

- Top with feta cheese crumbles and a bit of grated fresh Parmesan cheese

Bake covered at 375° for one hour. Uncover and sprinkle with grated Parmesan; bake an additional fifteen minutes uncovered.

Enchiladas

Preheat oven to 350°F.

On low-carb multigrain tortilla, spread thin layer of refried beans (make sure no lard is in the beans) then sprinkle finely chopped broccoli, grated cheddar, some fresh tomato, and a splash of enchilada sauce. Add soy crumbles if you would like a "meaty" flavor. Use part of enchilada sauce to cover bottom of 9"x13" glass baking dish; place rolled tortillas in the dish;

pour salsa or more enchilada sauce over the top to totally coat rolled tortillas. Bake at 350° for about thirty minutes. Sprinkle with more grated cheddar and bake until cheese is melted.

Skinny Cow

Blend together one scoop of vanilla protein mix (my choice is Pure Protein), two-thirds cup vanilla Soy Slender, a few drops of Vanilla Sweet Leaf Liquid Stevia, three or four ice cubes, and about a half cup diet root beer for a yummy, low-carb shake. Try a diet orange soft drink for a creamsicle flavor.

Resources

Lifestyle Resources
Medical and Personal Resources and
References
Running Resources
Swimming Resources
Highly Recommended Reading

Lifestyle Resources

Athletic and Lifestyle Apparel

www.underarmour.com

I live in UA tights year-round. Heat Gear in summer, Cold Gear in winter. I walked 35,000 miles since January 1, 2003 in Under Armor tights, leaving 150 pounds in my wake. The BEST athletic wear and gear on the planet. Period. Nothing more to say.

Food

www.costco.com

A good 90% of the food I ate to lose weight and now eat to keep it all off comes from Costco.

Walker's Hats

www.walkershatshop.com

Incredibly customizable selection of washable sun-protection hats and visors. I go for the biggest brims. And as one of my favorite former Chicago aldermen once told me, "Go big or go home!"

Jaw Bone UP

jawbone.com/up?r=awup10&gclid=CO_drvDCiroCFQkSMwoddQYA4Q

"Know Yourself, Live Better," is their slogan. UP™ is like a step counter and your conscience all rolled into one. UP's a wristband and app system that takes a holistic approach to a healthy lifestyle. The wristband tracks your movement and sleep in the background. The app displays your data, lets you add things like meals and mood, and delivers insights that keep you moving forward. UP then helps you use that information to work toward feeling your best.

A few of my guy pals swear by this neat little wristband and app system to help keep them on track. If I were just beginning my weight loss and wellness quest today, I'd race to get one of these babies. You should, too.

Digital Step Counter

www.digiwalker.com

Accurate. Long-lasting. I logged almost every one of my 35,000 walking miles wearing one of these. Back in 2002 it was just about the only one on the market that was highly accurate and built to last. I've given them as gifts and incentives to people I coach. Gift yourself with one.

Your Walking and Athletic Shoe Needs

www.holabirdsports.com

If you have a consistent favorite brand and model of athletic shoe, Holabird Sports has it for the best price. The same goes for all racquet sport items. The two and three-day shipping is free and they offer free returns for many items. How can you beat that? I just reorder a new pair of Brooks Adrenaline or Ariels every three months when I'm logging forty-five to fifty miles a week on average (You know I have shoe issues.). And please do tell them and their marketing director, Doug Crusse, that Laura Dion-Jones sent you.

Moji, the Smart Icing Alternative

www.gomoji.com

High performance recovery for your sore knees, Moji's products make icing more effective and comfortable by providing targeted cooling and full mobility. Moji's Cold Compression System—the most advanced cold therapy technology on the market—allows you to walk around while you ice. Just strap on the cold-cell knee wrap (made of high performance stretch fabric) and away you go. Moji also makes an incredible wrap for your back as well as a Thermos-like canister for traveling.

Those of you who know me and my chronic spine, leg, and knee pain issues know I live with ice packs on most of the time. Moji's are the bomb, and you can keep the packs on until they're not cold anymore. None of this so many minutes on and so many minutes off stuff, and there's no danger of frostbite with Moji ice packs. Visit their website for more expert icing, recovery, and training tips. Great website. Fabulous product. Designed by a female orthopedic surgeon—wouldn't you know it?

The Sole of Performance

www.sofsole.com

A moldable performance shoe footbed insert providing personalized fit and spectacular comfort. The next best thing to a custom-made orthotic—which I have lived in for half my life, so trust me. This one's much more cost effective in our current economy if you don't have any really special, horrid, physical issues with your back, legs, and feet. Follow the directions for heating them in your oven and customize by putting in your shoes and standing on them for a few minutes till they cool and mold to your feet.

Wildmind Buddhist Meditation

www.wildmind.org

Absolutely excellent beginner's Buddhist Breathing Meditation. A great way to start meditating. You can even do it where you're sitting right now—at your desk. It's not recommended to listen or practice meditation while driving. Try this one only at home.

Shapewear and Intimate Apparel

www.lipoinabox.com

Just what it sounds like: Lipo in a Box. "We make you look good with your clothes on." How can you go wrong with a motto like that? Tell the owner/founder Connie Elder that Laura Dion-Jones sent you. Her shapewear is the bomb and beats out that other S-word one: Spanx.

www.maidenform.com

Try their line of Fat Free Dressing˚ compression garments.

Canine Custom Performance Clothing and Accessories

www.snobhounds.com

"Think Nike meets Donna Karan, but for canines. True environmental protection wear with a Chanel twist." (Regardless of what Jay Leno says.) Guaranteed to keep your pooch warm, dry, cool, and comfy while walking with you, no matter what the weather.

Woodway Treadmills

www.woodway.com/

Woodway Treadmills save my back, knees, legs, hips, feet, ankles, and, above all, my spine, from the constant repetitive motion of other treadmills. CRM is deadly to any of us with special structural needs. So this is the one and only treadmill I will even consider using indoors. Thankfully for me, out of the 450 pieces of various state-of-the-art equipment in the cavernous cardio room at Chicago's East Bank Club, there are about eight of these beauties. Here's hoping they get more.

Rowing Machine

www.concept2.com/

If I had the room in my house and needed to have an incredible fat-burning machine, this would be the one. Check into their refurbished models, if you're so inclined.

All my doctors tell me that this is the most overlooked but most important piece of cardio equipment in the club because it works practically every muscle in your entire body—and that's a really good thing. If you're putting in the time, why not move all your limbs at once, instead of just half of them?

Schwinn Airdyne

www.schwinnfitness.com/schwinn_fitness_us/homepage.jsp

Another terrific non-weight-bearing cardio machine guaranteed to keep you sweatin' to the oldies while all four limbs move in time to your tunes.

NuStep Recumbent Climber

www.nustep.com/us/professional

Have a hankering to climb Mt. Everest or just shed some unhealthy, unwanted weight? Start right here. The NuStep is a recumbent climber that works all four limbs at once. By regulating the intensity of the resistance from one to ten, this baby will kick butt in no time. Don't let the "old lady rehab machine" connotation fool you. I've seen grown men cry, or maybe it was just sweat rolling down their cheeks, when working at a level ten. Start slow. Steady as you go. You'll get there. Everest can't be climbed in a day, either.

Dance Your Way to Better Health

My two Dance Mavens who help me achieve better balance, movement, flexibility and clarity through dance. I could not live without them. What more could you ask for – extra cardio disguised as dance!

Tommye Giacchino
US & World Champion Ballroom Dancer
T.Giacchino@Icloud.com
www.windycityweddingdance.com

And:

Lisa "La Boriqua"
Founder, Latin Street Dancing
President & Director, Latin Street Dance Academy
Latin Dance Visionary
1335 W Lake St, Ste 103
Chicago, IL 60607
312-42-SALSA * 312-427-2572
www.LatinStreetDancing.com

Medical Resources and Personal References

"No man is fit to command another who cannot command himself."

—William Penn, seventeenth century British religious leader and founder
of Pennsylvania

The advice contained in this book is provided for motivational purposes only. It is based on my extensive, personal (and sometimes painful) experience and research in diet, fitness, beauty, and fashion. I have the equivalent of a Ph.D. in Obesity, having lived a lifetime in chronic obesity's shoes.

The information in the book is not intended as a substitute for a medically supervised diet plan. The ideas and methods I put forth are my opinion, based on what has worked for me, and do not necessarily reflect the opinions of the doctors and health care providers who are part of my personal health and fitness team. I include them here as personal references because they did what I feel health care professionals should do: they treated me like an individual and helped me develop diet, health, and fitness methods that work for me and can work for you, too.

My incredible 150-pound weight loss is the result of intense self-motivation, developing discipline, daily fitness walking, and the careful contributions of all of these gifted professionals. Each has greatly impacted my well-being and physical and personal appearance, when so many others I consulted either could not or would not. I am where I am today in part because of them, and I am lucky to be able to call each of them a friend.

If the diet, health, and fitness plan you currently follow is not working for you, please question every professional with whom you're working. It is your responsibility to carefully consider what diet, medical, health, and fitness advice you choose to follow or reject. Find the right doctors and/or health care providers for you—the ones who will work with you on your terms. Tell them what's working for you and what's not, and go forward from there. When it comes to your health care and the professionals you choose to work with, remember: It's your money. It's your body. It's your life.

Keep searching until you get the positive results you desire. It has taken me a lifetime to achieve the healthy lifestyle I have now, and I feel compelled to share my success with everyone who is in need of a motivational best friend. I can certainly help make you over into the new person your old person only dreams of being, beginning with improving your health and losing weight by finding the diet that's right for you and by walking your way to wellness.

I'm always here for you in any way I can be. Just call or e-mail me.

James Hill, M.D.
Professor of Orthopedic Surgery
Department of Orthopedic Surgery
Northwestern University
675 N. St. Clair Street
Suite 17-100
Chicago, IL 60611
Tel 312-695-6800
Fax 312-695-0236

This man is truly a god among men and one of the most gifted, brilliant, sincere, and unassuming human beings you'll ever meet. He saved my right leg after a hideous skiing accident many years ago and today I walk daily largely because of him. (He was the eighth doctor I consulted within the week immediately following my ski accident. Doctor number seven and number eight concurred on the course of my treatment; I chose Dr. Hill.)

Mark Stolar, M.D.
Associate Professor of Clinical Medicine
Division of Endocrinology
Northwestern University
Northwestern Internists, Ltd.
676 N. St. Clair Street
Suite 415
Chicago, IL 60611
Tel 312-335-1133
Fax 312-335-9774
Chicago, IL

Another god among men. He listened, he never prejudged, and he took steps to help me find myself where none other could or would. I am forever grateful. Dr. Stolar was probably the sixth doctor I went to over the course of several years for weight loss and wellness help. Second, third, and even fourth opinions do count; they help you find the right way to wellness for you.

Julius Few, M.D.
The Few Institute for Aesthetic Plastic Surgery
875 N. Michigan Avenue, Suite #3850
Chicago, IL 60611
Tel 312-202-0882
www.fewinstitute.com
2013-Present: Health System Clinician, Northwestern Memorial Hospital
2008-Present: Clinical Associate, Division of Plastic Surgery, University of Chicago

2000-2008: Assistant and Associate Professor, Division of Plastic Surgery, Northwestern University Feinberg School of Medicine

The third god in the triumvirate, Dr. Few has worked miracles with my body that I never thought possible: tummy tuck, new and improved belly button, breast lift, and underarm and inner thigh lifts—and it's not over yet.

Colleen M. Fitzgerald, MD, MS
Associate Professor
Loyola University Medical Center
Department of Obstetrics and Gynecology
Division of Uro-gynecology, Pelvic Medicine
2160 S. First Ave.
Maywood, IL 60153
Appts: 708-216-2180
Assistant: Frankie Bailey 708-216-2170
E-mail: cfitzgerald@lumc.edu

Goddess of "Detective Medicine," as I like to call her. She had the tenacity to get to the bottom of my chronic nerve pain and pinpoint arachnoiditis of the spine. If not for her, I'd still be pursuing every fad treatment in the book without knowing why none would work for me. She helped me channel my strength and fitness efforts to hang onto what physical abilities I have left and then build upon that, which I work on every single day.

Cynthia E. Caldarella, D.C.
Chiropractic Physician
The Wellness Studio
1731 N. Marcey St., Suite 530
Chicago, IL 60614
Tel (312) 852-7850

Education:

B.S. in psychology, University of Iowa

B.S. in general science, National College of Chiropractic (Now known as National University of Health Sciences)

Dr. of Chiropractic, National College of Chiropractic (Now known as National University of Health Sciences)

Ten months ago, I had steroid shots in my cervical and lumbar spine for some of my chronic pain issues. I traditionally get these injections twice a year and had the last ones in June 2012, and they worked like the proverbial charm. This last series I received worked their magic for about a week.

It was heaven being totally pain free. Then, for whatever reason, they backfired and I was left to deal with incredible pain that was off the charts. The shots aggravated, instead of soothed, my spinal condition. I was never more miserable in my life. Nothing, nothing, nothing I tried worked. A friend recommended I see chiropractor, Dr. Cynthia Caldarella, to help manage the pain and also get me on the road to a more holistic way of wellness.

I have to say that Dr. C. worked her butt off to help me. My improvement was slow, but steady. Now she helps me manage my chronic pain without steroids or shots. Dr. C. is quite a wonderful addition to my medical support team and I am proud to also call her a friend.

Jackie Detry, CMT
Certified Pilates Trainer
Certified Gyrokinesis/Gyrotonics Trainer
East Bank Club
500 N. Kingsbury Street
Chicago, IL 60654

While I was losing weight and developing my daily walking regimen, I knew I needed something more to help me get stronger and manage my chronic pain more effectively. The meager weight training I was doing at the time clearly wasn't enough. Then I discovered Pilates and Jackie Detry. Jackie is a master of her craft; I like to call her my "Pilates Therapist" because of what she did for me. I took six years of weekly private lessons with Jackie, and we then added Gyrotonics, a vital addition to balance my weekly fitness routine. I can't say enough about Pilates, Gyrotoncis, and Jackie Detry. They all help strengthen my core.

Julie O'Connell, PT

Performing Arts Medicine Manager
Athletico Physical Therapy
East Bank Club
500 N. Kingsbury Street
Chicago, IL 60654
Tel 312-527-5801 ext.278

Julie was athletic trainer for the U.S. Women's Olympic Soccer Team (Greece) and artistic trainer for The Joffrey Ballet, Hubbard Street Dance Company, and many other top dance companies across the country. Dr. James Hill, my orthopedic surgeon, sent me to Julie, Supreme Goddess of the PT World, to stave off a total knee replacement for as long as possible. (See the following on Dr. Stulberg.)

I scoffed. I whined. I moaned and dragged my feet because I didn't understand what miracles and healing power physical therapy had until Julie got her hands on me—literally. She worked my bones, muscles, and frame like no one else ever did. She twisted, pulled, elbowed, yanked, and prodded my crooked leg and other structural issues to make me straighter and stronger in every way possible. When I remarked how much her ministrations had improved my walking and how much stronger I was, she replied, "You're in command of the ground now, the ground is no longer in command of you." She wasn't kidding.

Erin Weinhardt, PT, DPT
Athletico Physical Therapy
East Bank Club
Assistant Facility Manager
Physical Therapist
500 N. Kingsbury St.
Chicago, IL 60654
Tel 312-527-5801 x 278
Fax 312-644-4567

During this last go-around with my spine pain flare, Erin stepped in to help me with more PT, under instruction and direction from Dr. Cynthia Calderella. It helps when your doctor and PT are on the same page. There are no excuses and these two gals really help me get through my days, enabling me to practice what I teach.

Dr. S. David Stulberg
Northwestern Orthopaedic Institute
680 N. Lake Shore Drive, Suite #924
Chicago, IL 60611
Tel 312-664-6848
Professor of Orthopaedic Surgery, Northwestern University Feinberg School of Medicine
Founder and director of the Joint Reconstruction and Implant Service at Northwestern Memorial Hospital

Dr. Stulberg is a member of the Hip Society and the Knee Society of America, a cofounder of the International Society for Technology in Arthoplasty, a founding member of the International Society for Computer Assisted Orthopaedic Surgery, a fellow of the American Academy of Orthopaedic Surgery, a member of the Board of Directors of Rehabilitation Institute of Chicago, and is on staff at Rush North Shore Medical Center.

A pioneer in computer-assisted, minimally invasive surgical techniques, Dr. S. David Stulberg is universally recognized as being one of the world's top orthopaedic surgeons. He has taught, influenced, and inspired thousands of physicians and surgeons from all over the world.

Dr. Stulberg is especially proud of his leadership role with "Operation Walk Chicago," through which hundreds of total joint replacements are annually performed free of charge in disadvantaged areas throughout the world. In addition to his clinical work, Dr. Stulberg holds several patents on surgical instruments and is also a coauthor of books and hundreds of professional publications. He lectures frequently in America and abroad.

In June of 2009, I finally had to throw up the white flag and get a total right knee replacement. And, you know me, after doing all the research, and liking to go only to the best, I chose Dr. Stulberg to do the surgery. Boy, am I ever glad I did. I now have a straight right leg for the first time in the nearly twenty years since my hideous skiing accident, and I can walk better than I did the day before the surgery.

On March 31, 2011, Dr. Stulberg replaced my left knee, which became the crooked one after the right knee was replaced. I couldn't imagine what it was going to be like with two straight legs and about 150 pounds less of me to haul around on them. Now I know.

The sky's the limit! And for you, too!

James R. Bailes, Jr., M.D., F.A.A.P.
Pediatric Endocrinology
Specializing in childhood obesity
Associate Professor of Pediatrics
Marshall University School of Medicine
1600 Medical Center Drive, Suite #3500
Huntington, WV 25701
Tel 304-691-1300

Coauthor of *No More Fat Kids: A Pediatrician's Guide For Safe and Effective Weight Loss,* Dr. Bailes specializes in childhood obesity and has developed an incredibly successful weight loss program for school-aged children in which they lose weight without feeling hungry. The program improves overall health, lipid profiles, and, most importantly, self-esteem, and has changed the lives of hundreds of children. Dr. Bailes's straightforward, practical, and easy-to-follow approach will change the life of your child, too. I'm glad he's now a friend and on my professional medical advisory team.

The chapter on Insulin and the Carbohydrate Factor in this book is taken directly from Dr. Jamie's book, *No More Fat Kids: A Pediatrician's Guide For Safe and Effective Weight Loss* with his kind permission, because I wanted to give you the simplest, most comprehensive explanation about this subject that I had available and Dr. Jamie explains it in very simple, understandable terms.

I told Jamie that his book should be titled *No More Fat People* because it's written for kids but encompasses everyone's health and fitness regardless of age and could help put an end to our country's obesity epidemic.

Colette Heimowitz, M.Sc.
VP Nutrition & Education
Atkins Nutritionals, Inc.
Center for Research and Development Quality
370 E. Maple Avenue, Suite 301
Langhorne, PA 19047
Tel 303-395-0973

A longtime supporter of my cause and the "Maven of Low-Carb Dieting," Colette jokes that I know more about the Atkins Diet at "the street level," than they do. And since I continue to live a modified Atkins lifestyle—to the best of my ability, even with constant temptation—to maintain my weight. For the first time in my entire life, I've managed to hang onto my 150-pound weight loss for ten years, when before I had zoomed right back up the scale. I'm proud to have Colette on my Professional Advisory Team, too.

Myles Harston
AquaRanch Industries
PO Box 658
Flannagan, IL 61740
Tel 309-208-5230
www.aquaranch.com

Myles is the country's foremost authority and supplier of totally organic, hydroponic, and aquaponics systems, supplies, and equipment. He also grows and sells his incredible organic produce and farm-raised, hormone-free tilapia to restaurants and stores all around the Chicagoland area. Once you've tasted Myles's fresh, organic produce and fish, it's difficult to eat anything else. His lettuce tastes like lettuce used to taste back when we were kids, before all the pesticides, preservatives, and additives. Myles cultivates and raises the only hormone-free, organic tilapia in the country and once you taste his, you won't even look at the fish raised in Thailand, China, or anywhere else.

Myles is also on my Professional Advisory team because no one on earth knows more about aquaculture, hydroponics, organic farming, and organic fish farming, as well as ethanol and all of the other environmental hazards out there. He's literally a walking encyclopedia on all things healthy, sustainable, organic, and environmentally sound.

Dr. Clare M. Ollayos, DC
30 N. Airlite Street, Suite C
Elgin, IL 60123
Tel 847-888-9988

Dr. Clare took care of all my chiropractic needs when I had my talk radio show in Elgin, Illinois. She's a terrific chiropractor and especially gifted with acupuncture, helping me manage my chronic pain in a very holistic, gentle way.

Dr. Eleanor (Elly) Laser, Ph.D.
Cell 312 961 7727
www.laserhypnosis.com

Dr. Elly uses the hypnosis technique "Sweet Tooth Extraction" to help those of us who are hopelessly, chronically addicted to sweets, no matter how low-carb we eat. Once an addict, always an addict, I always say. It's all in how you manage your addiction, isn't it? Elly helped me manage my chocolate addiction by "extracting my sweet tooth."

Dr. Sergey Sokolov, DN
Naprapath
NES & Bioresonance Professional
Professional Track & Field Coach
Sergey51@live.com
Cell 847-708-9562

Sergey is my ultimate PT—the Physical Therapist & Personal Trainer I cannot live without. He and I work together every Thursday morning for forty-five minutes; part of that time he works on my soft tissue and using Thai massage, stretching, and other modalities, then we work on strength and balance techniques that I practice every single day right after my minimum of an hour's cardio. If you have physical issues like I do and refuse to let them stop you in your tracks on your way to healthier weight loss and improved fitness, you have to see a very good, qualified physical therapist/personal trainer. Your health and well-being depend on it. And if you practice daily what they teach you in your sessions, you'll move and groove much better.

~ ~ ~

Not a day goes by that I don't have some sort of chronic pain issue to deal with that could, if I let it, stop me from taking another step on that daily walk of life. I refuse to let it. I have diligently worked with my medical team to identify my physical problems and challenges, what to do about them, and how I can keep walking daily through all of it.

Not walking daily is *not* an option for me—it's *that* important.

I hope you'll be motivated to do the same.

Running Resources*

Organizations and Groups

American Running Association: www.americanrunning.org

Road Runners Club of America: www.rrca.org

Professional Road Running Organization: www.prro.org

American Trail Running Association:
www.trailrunner.com/links/running_organizations.htm

Run Diva: www.rundiva.net/running-clubs-organizations/

Running Equipment and Accessories

Holabird Sports: www.holabirdsports.com

Road Runner Sports: www.roadrunnersports.com

Gear.com: www.gear.com/s/running/

Magazines

Runners World Magazine: www.runnersworld.com

Women's Running Magazine: www.womensrunning.competitor.com/

Trail Runner Magazine: www.trailrunnermag.com

Running Times Magazine: www.runningtimes.com/running-times

* URLs may change at any time.

Swimming Resources*

Organizational Groups and Programs

U.S. Masters Swimming: www.usms.org

USA Swimming: www.usaswimming.org

USA Swimming - local swimming committees/clubs by state: www.usaswimming.org/DesktopDefault.aspx(scroll down and click on Find a Club on the left side of the page)

Swim America – Learn to Swim Programs: www.swimamerica.org

YMCA: ymca.net/swim-sports-play

International Swimming Federation: www.fina.org

American Red Cross (Swimming & Water Safety): www.redcross.org/take-a-class/program-highlights/swimming

Swimming Needs & Accessories

Arena: www.arenausa.com

Speedo USA: www.speedousa.com

TYR: www.tyr.com

USA Swimming Store: http://shop.usaswimming.org/

Swim Outlet: www.swimoutlet.com

Magazines

Splash Magazine: hard copy or online at
www.nxtbook.com/nxtbooks/usaswimming/splash_20130708/index.php

Swimming World Magazine: www.swimmingworldmagazine.com

FINA Aquatics World Magazine:
www.fina.org/H2O/index.php?option=com_content&view=article&id=142
8&Itemid=374

*URLs may change at any time.

Highly Recommended Reading

It's strictly up to you to educate yourself about your own health and fitness. Knowledge is power. Use it to your advantage. In my opinion, the following is a list of some of the most important health, fitness, and diet books you can read, other than mine:

1. *Dr. Atkins' New Diet Revolution. The Amazing No-Hunger Weight Loss Plan That Has Helped Millions Lose Weight and Keep It Off* by Robert C. Adkins, M.D.

I'm living proof that this diet (in a modified form for me) not only works, it is safe and can be used to maintain your weight loss and wellness long term, regardless of what some of the "experts" say.

You gotta wanna, and if you really wanna, you'll find the right way that works for you. See if you can get your hands on a copy.

2. *The NEW Atkins For A New You, The ULTIMATE DIET for SHEDDING WEIGHT and FEELING GREAT* by Dr. Eric C. Westman, Dr. Stephen D. Phinney, and Dr. Jeff S. Volek.

This book is backed by today's science of over fifty studies and redesigned to help you lose weight fast and stay lean for life. It features personalized meal plans, all-new recipes, and inspiring success stories. How would you like to lose fifteen pounds in two weeks. You can with the Atkins low-carb way of life.

3. *No More Fat Kids: A Pediatrician's Guide For Safe and Effective Weight Loss*, by Dr. James R. Bailes, Jr., M.D., with Dr. Misty Trent-Strow, M.D..

An eye-opener of a book, this is a comprehensive guide to improving an overweight child's overall health, well-being, and self-esteem. As an adult reading his book, I found that it helped clarify and demystify the principles of a safe, healthy low-carb diet and lifestyle. Dr. Jamie simply explains the impact that an overproduction of insulin has on our system and what we can do about it. I told Dr. Jamie that he should've titled his book *No More Fat People,* because it will help everyone understand the safe, effective, healthy low-carb way of life in plain, simple language.

4. *Good Calories. Bad Calories: Challenging the Conventional Wisdom on Diet, Weight Control, and Disease* by Gary Taubes.

Another eye-opener of a book. I wish every physician, dietician, and health care professional in the world would put ego aside and read this one. It might enable the ones still clinging to outdated diet dogma to help you more effectively by pointing out important evidence of another viable option rather than the same old, same old.

If you find this book a bit of a technical slog, search the *New York Times* database for his eight-page article of the same title. Think of it as the "CliffsNotes" of his book.

5. The Zone: A Revolutionary Life Plan to Put Your Body in Total Balance for Permanent Weight Loss by Barry Sears, Ph.D.

One of my former doctors pooh-poohed this diet when I wanted to go on it while under his care several years ago. I went ahead and did it anyway since the diet he prescribed didn't work for me at all, and six weeks later, much to his surprise and mine, my LDL and HDL were a good sixty-some points lower and my triglycerides experienced a significant decline. When I pointed all this out to him, he said it was "a fluke." I said, "Adios." Then I found Dr. Mark Stolar. Case in point: When in doubt, always, always, always get another opinion.

6. *The South Beach Diet* by Arthur Agatston, M.D.

Very Atkins-like, but drawn out in a slightly different manner. Some like this diet because of the "South Beach-y" glamour aspect of it. Too broad-based for me, however. I need a more Atkins-like approach. Whatever works, do it.

7. *The Diabetes Carbohydrate and Fat Gram Guide* by Lea Ann Holzmeister, RD, CDE, is a handy reference guide to count your carbs accurately.

A comprehensive carbohydrate and fat gram counting guide like the one Atkins has is an excellent resource, as well. I highlight and flag all my favorite foods and refer to both books often.

Programs and Seminars

Laura's Commit To Get Fit programs and support seminars will help you find the secret to your own true and everlasting weight loss once and for all. Commit To Get Fit is a no-nonsense, comprehensive approach to a fit and healthy lifestyle for individuals, organizations, or workplace wellness programs. Commit To Get Fit was developed by Certified Corporate Wellness Coach (CCWC) and Certified Wellness Coach (CWC) Laura Dion-Jones, who turned a lifetime of chronic obesity into weight-loss success. It's not a quick fix, but a proven, easy-to-follow weight-loss program that really works.

Whether you're ten, twenty, fifty, or 100 pounds or more overweight, you can reach and maintain a healthier weight for life with the Commit To Get Fit motivational weight-loss and wellness programs. Laura's approach is a blend of accountability-based weight loss management, fitness programs, and motivational seminars, but her programs are tailored to the needs of individuals (and groups) for healthy, sustainable weight loss.

Laura also works with companies that are dedicated to their employees' health. Highlighting key components of her own weight-loss success, Laura will help you and your employees achieve the same type of results she achieved. She'll help you find the diet that's right for you, develop walking into a daily lifelong healthy cardio habit, and learn to make healthier food choices you can live with through holidays, birthdays, and beyond.

Laura's high-energy presentations and accountability-based coaching style helps individuals achieve short-, medium-, and long-term goals through critical, actionable steps. This works because most people need a combination of education, behavior change, accountability, and encouragement to achieve healthy and sustainable weight loss.

Laura's hugely successful "Commit To Get Fit/Elgin's Biggest Loser" motivational weight loss and wellness program, which she held through her weekly talk radio show on WRMN 1410 AM, helped motivate many, many Elgin and Fox Valley area residents to lose hundreds and hundreds of pounds. Let Laura help you, your employees, or members of your organization become happier, healthier, and more fit!

See www.commit-fit.com for more details and information on various programs and seminars, and to find out how Laura can help you, your company, group, or organization Commit To Get Fit once and for all.

Rates and program details available upon request.

About the Author

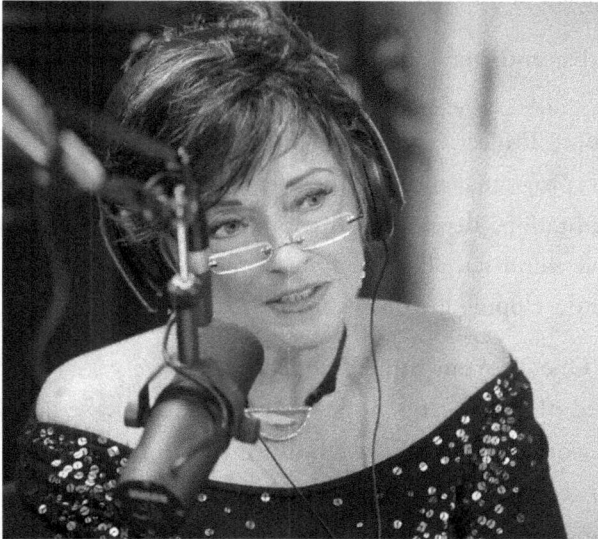

Laura Dion-Jones is a Pro-Health Activist, Certified Corporate Wellness Coach (CCWC), Certified Wellness Coach (CWC), highly sought after TV and radio show host, motivational and lifestyle writer, professional speaker, and author.

People say that Laura has the equivalent of a Ph.D. in Obesity, having lived in those shoes for most of her life. There is nothing anyone can tell her about being obese that she doesn't already know firsthand.

In addition, Laura's extensive background in the fashion and beauty industries led her to become one of the nation's first and top plus-size designers with Dion-Jones, Ltd., from 1986-1998 (www.dionjonesltd.com). She has hundreds of successful personal appearance makeovers for women, as well as men, to her credit.

Laura was also one of the nation's first and top plus-size models from 1980-1998, appearing in numerous TV commercials as well as newspaper and magazine ads from Bloomingdale's, Bergdorf's, Marshall Field's, Saks Fifth Avenue, and Sears, to I. Magnin, K-Mart, Venture, and Zayre, to name but a few—way back in the day.

Her innovative and highly successful "Commit To Get Fit With Laura Dion-Jones," her "Chicago High School Teens and Teachers Transformation Project," and her "Elgin's Biggest Loser Competition" motivational programs and support seminars teach the basics of daily walking, meditation, developing discipline, maximizing human potential, and a positive mind-set, all while finding the right diet and fitness routine necessary for developing lifelong change.

Laura is a "One Woman Straight Eye for the Every Gal or Every Guy" who's in need of a motivational best friend to help make people over into the new person they have always dreamed of being. Her tough love motivational techniques raise people's awareness of lifestyle choices so that they can take control of their weight, their fitness, their appearance, their self-esteem, and their lives.

Laura sells people on themselves and ultimately makes them believe that if she can do it, they most certainly can, too. And then she shows them how …

While not as heavy-handed as TV's "Biggest Loser," Laura's programs are accountability-based, which means they require a little weekly reading; keeping weight, cardio, and food logs; and attending weekly weigh-ins and support group meetings that comprise her seminars.

An avid urban hiker who is known to average forty-eight to fifty-five miles a week, she can be seen walking around Chicago's Gold Coast, Magnificent Mile, River North, and downtown areas, most of the time with her two little Italian Greyhounds in tow. Laura is now considered an Elite Walker by many marathoners because she walks more miles in a week than most train. Learn more about Laura and her weight-loss coaching services at her website www.commit-fit.com/index.php and her blog at www.commit-fit.blogspot.com/.

P.S.: Please send Laura your own weight-loss and personal success stories for a future book: laura@commit-fit.com. You will be in a position to help many others through your own struggles and triumphs.

The Laura Dion-Jones – Commit To Get Fit Foundation, a 501(c)3 NFP

Laura started her foundation to make her Commit To Get Fit seminars, programs, and books available to all, regardless of socio or economic situations.

Her goal is to have Commit To Get Fit With Laura Dion-Jones provide accountability-based fitness programs and motivational seminars with a variety of approaches tailored to the needs of participants and individuals for healthy weight loss, fostering a culture of wellness within a company, community, organization, or on an individual basis. This wellness environment energizes and empowers people and employees to become healthier and more fit, which results in better health and beneficial bottom-line savings for all.

Laura's Vision:

Laura's vision is to combat our country's escalating obesity epidemic by creating awareness and building healthier companies and communities through redefining and improving the healthy eating and fitness of all individuals with an emphasis on health, wellness, and behavior change.

By educating people about healthier diet and daily cardio options they may not have thought of or even tried before, Laura makes sure her clients and seminar participants know they have choices: other options in diet, health, fitness and lifestyle than they're traditionally used to.

The Mission:

Laura gives people courage and hope when and where there is none by proving positive change is possible and that the rewards are immediate—all they have to do is want to improve their health and fitness and meet her halfway. She then shows them how to begin with the first steps that carry them through till they reach their weight loss and fitness goals. But they're not done yet; Laura then shows them how to maintain their new health and fitness levels for the rest of their lives.

The How:

Laura's C2GF coaching interactions touch on the physical, emotional, and environmental aspects of each person or employee's life by taking a comprehensive approach to promoting lifestyle change for improved health.

Laura helps her C2GF clients and seminar participants find the diet that's right for them, develop daily cardio discipline, and achieve lifelong wellness success by building on skills which will carry on through other parts of the participants' lives.

Laura says, "You gotta wanna, there is no other way," then she helps people wanna and shows them how.

The Method:

Physical health includes nutrition, strength training, and meditation to rest, relax, and reset our minds and strengthen our willpower and resolve.

By taking past and present injuries and illnesses into consideration, Laura helps people improve their weight, cholesterol, blood pressure, and the rest of their biometric numbers through education and leading by example. Laura not only walks the walk, but walks the talk having lost 130 pounds in two and a half years on her own—no gimmicks, no fads, and with a severe disability from a ski injury that has been currently corrected through two knee replacements but still requires daily vigilance in the form of a low-carb diet, daily cardio, and various strength training and physical therapy modalities.

The Laura Dion-Jones - Commit To Get Fit Foundation accepts financial support from individuals and corporate entities to further its mission in making her Commit To Get Fit seminars, programs, and books available to everyone who needs them, regardless of their ability to pay. Your support in funding Laura's C2GF Foundation would be greatly appreciated. Please contact Laura directly for information on how to donate: laura@commit-fit.com.

Acknowledgements

* Special thanks to my editors, graphic artists, formatter, publicist, IT boys, coaches, and all my friends and support personnel for their help in developing this book. One simply cannot do this kind of thing alone.

* Another special thanks to all my doctors and medical and fitness professionals who helped me get healthy and continue to help me stay this way.

* To all my original Elgin's Biggest Losers: You each had a hand in helping me help motivate you, and you contributed to formulating my *Commit To Get Fit* book, programs, and seminar series as they are now. I gave you the weight loss and wellness tools that will help you lose and keep your weight off forever, if you wanna; what you do with them is strictly up to you. Just know that you no longer have any excuses. It was my sincere pleasure working with each one of you. I am profoundly changed, immensely humbled and forever indebted.

* To my "Kids": my class of eight extremely exceptional young people who made up my mentoring group through The Elgin Youth Leadership Academy's (YLA) Service Learning Project. As an adult student participant of The Elgin Leadership Academy and Service Learning Project, I was asked to be a mentor to eight at-risk youth from YLA. My topic was nutrition, and I was lucky enough to have eight of the most exceptional young people I've ever had the pleasure to meet and work with in my coaching care.

I split the kids into four teams of two each, helped them select their different diet dogma topics from the four most popular weight loss plans, directed and encouraged them, and let them go to town with the research and PowerPoint presentation we ultimately presented to Elgin's brand new Mayor, Dave Kaptain, at his first Elgin Town Council Meeting in May of 2011. (I encouraged my kids to shoot for the stars. If we're gonna present, let's present where it really counts.) Subsequently, I had the Elgin Town

Council presentation footage and the kids' PowerPoint presentation made into a mini documentary of the same title: *Dear Mrs. Obama: To End Our Country's Obesity Epidemic, Please Redefine Healthy Eating.* It can be found at www.dearmrsobama.com.

* To Otis Wilson – for being the first to notice I was losing weight way back in the beginning. Otis came up to me one day at EBC and said, "Hey, Baby, you look like you're losing weight!"

"Yeah, I am! Thanks for noticing!" I exclaimed. I had lost my *first* five pounds, down from 317.

Otis, you were the very first to notice. Thanks for the encouragement, Pal.

* To Noah "You can't exercise away a bad diet" Richter. Former Ace Personal Trainer at Chicago's East Bank Club. Thanks for being my Rent-a-Son. I couldn't have asked for more.

* To Devon Polderman – for your exceptional insight, guidance, and teaching me the importance of story.

* To Paula Babcock who encouraged me to write this book to help others do what I did and put an end to our country's obesity epidemic - once and for all.

* To Tommye Giacchino, International and National Ballroom Champion, and Lisa "La Boriqua" of Latin Street Dance Academy, two of the top dance instructors in Chicago, for helping me achieve better balance, movement and clarity through dance.

* Tony Laban - for your invaluable help ...

* To MF – you know why.

* To MAB – thank you for the lessons. You're responsible for what's coming next.

When a person tells you who they are, believe them.

* God bless you all. I am eternally grateful ...

The End

You can read the ending of this book first thing, thinking it's just like every other how-to, self-help, diet, and fitness book on the planet, and think you'll know the "secret to finding your own true and everlasting weight loss," but you won't "get it" until you actually sit down and read the entire book, using it as your guide to help formulate your own new, healthy lifestyle and fitness plan.

However, the real secret to finding your own true and everlasting weight loss is not here at the end, it's the steps you take on your journey along the way ...

You gotta wanna.

Good health and fitness all depend on how well you work your routine.

In the end, it *is* all up to you.

There is no other way.

Good luck.

XOXO,

Laura

Marilyn Tam, bestselling Author of "The Happiness Choice," Speaker, former CEO of Aveda, President of Reebok Apparel Products & Retail Group, and VP of Nike.

Laura Dion-Jones walks her talk. Read and benefit from her journey from fat to fab. Laura is down to earth, funny, and wise from practical experience and research on what truly works in regaining and maintaining a healthy body. You'll love her book, so get it. You and your body will thank you for it.

Otis Wilson, #55, Former Chicago Bear football player and Super Bowl Champ:

"It was good seeing you work so hard. Congratulations. You rock! Keep up the good work."

Mikki Williams, CSP, CPAE:

She's a fitness ninja, a nutrition warrior, a glamour gal, a creative entrepreneur, a captivating coach, a motivational powerhouse, and a passionate and compassionate champion of everyone achieving their health, fitness and weight loss goals. Now you can share in her wisdom and her commitment and achieve all that she has. Laura Dion-Jones is the only "diet pill" that works!!!

Colette Heimowicz, M.Sc., VP Nutrition & Education, Atkins Nutritionals, Inc.:

Laura gives us a straight from the hip approach that will change the way you approach food and exercise. She is an inspiration for those who struggle with food. Follow her advice and it will change the way you look, how you feel, and how long you live.

Mark Stolar, M.D., Associate Professor of Clinical Medicine, Division of Endocrinology, *Northwestern University, Northwestern Internists, Ltd.*:

So many "experts" in the weight management field talk but don't walk the path to fitness and wellness. Laura's commitment to fitness and wellness is remarkable, not only personally but in helping others commit to get fit in a balanced and sustainable way.

James R. Bailes, Jr., M.D., F.A.A.P., Pediatric Endocrinology, Specializing in childhood obesity, Associate Professor of Pediatrics, Marshall University School of Medicine:

Laura Dion-Jones knows weight loss! She has personally experienced every diet imaginable and figured out that a reduced carbohydrate diet combined with daily exercise is easy to follow and successful! ! C2GF is a lifestyle plan that will change lives! This is as easy as it gets in the realm of diet and exercise.

Karyn Calabrese, The country's top vegan and raw food nutritionist:

As I often say, there are many roads to the top of the mountain and this is true for all aspects of our lives.

Laura certainly has a place for anyone in their healing and transformation process.

Baby steps work for many, some people can jump in 100% but that doesn't work for everyone. She certainly has found a process that works for her and can be passed down to many to help them improve at their own pace.

Love and gratitude for all you do,

Karyn

George Rawlinson, author and publisher.

I have worked with and known Laura Dion-Jones for several years. She has a unique and unparalleled perspective on health and fitness—a perspective that is incredible to hear. She is an encyclopedia of practical knowledge and a caring, compassionate motivational guide for readers who want to transform themselves into healthier, happier adults. Laura's ongoing mission is to be of service. I remain a friend and fan for life.

Read, listen, and learn!

Clare M. Ollayos, D.C.:

Laura has literally walked her talk. She has a no-nonsense, straightforward approach to health, focusing on both fitness and weight management. Importantly, her holistic approach involves healthy food choices, portion control, and finding an exercise combination that works and making it a lifestyle rather than a short-term fix. Many of her food choices are excellent for persons with gluten or dairy sensitivity as well. Read this book and enjoy more vitality!

Eleanor (Elly) Laser, PhD:

Laura Dion-Jones' book is a revelation about the struggle and discrimination the obese person goes through.

Laura climbed up a steep mountain, counting on herself to find the path leading to the top. Her ultimate weight loss success is an inspirational story illustrating that anyone can be helped.

Her theme throughout is never give up. She builds the reader's encouragement, which is the key to change.

I specialize in medical hypnosis. I am honored to have been one part of her successful outcome with the "Sweet Tooth Extraction."

Sue Koch, Strategic Social Media Coach and Speaker:

This book is a must read for anyone who thinks it cannot be done, who has succumbed to the idea that "this is just my lot in life." Laura did it against all odds, finding the path to success that even doctors could not afford her. Her candid yet caring writing style will draw you in and her authenticity will help you to feel understood where no one else could. She is the coach you've been seeking and will finally make you realize you can change your life, you can be healthy. Read it. Follow it. Commit to get fit with Laura!

Rickey Gold – Public Relations:

Laura writes in a smart, funny, honest, if-I-did-it-you-can-do-it style. Her books are fun to read because she's so warm, authentic, and a great storyteller. *Commit To Get Fit* is loaded with tips, motivation, and inspiration for achieving a healthy and fit lifestyle. Laura shares how she struggled for years until she finally discovered the key to weight loss and maintenance. The wisdom she shares in this book can help you lose weight and achieve a healthy lifestyle as well … whether you want to lose ten pounds or two hundred.

Testimonials

Kay Kosinski-Duren:

My first thought is "Action is the antidote to our sense of powerlessness, and Action is Laura's middle name. Just look at those words "Commit" and "Get Fit."Laura has lived action and she inspires through her experience. There is no better action one could take for oneself than to heed Laura's advice."

Kendra Span

Laura,

Just wanted to say thank you for the motivating workshop on Tuesday. I know what I need to do, it's just a matter of actually doing it on a consistent basis. I feel like I really "wanna" —it's pretty much all I think of every day. But I realize as a busy mom with 2 kids, working full time, I just put everyone else ahead of me and the result has been disastrous.

I'm just completely disgusted with my own excuses, my own failures, and disappointing myself over and over. I really liked the questions you posed, "How badly do I want it? What am I willing to give up? What commitments can I make?" I'm the only one stopping myself. "Deep down I know the right thing to do—the worst thing is to do nothing at all."

So here are my new DAILY goals.

Track all my food on MyFitnessPal app (tracks carbs too)

Limit carbs to 30 net carbs per day

Walk 1 hour every day (even Sunday)

Weigh myself every morning and log it

Take my Metformin every night

Get 8 hours of sleep every night

Thank you for your incredible support.

Kendra

Dear Laura:

I've enjoyed spending Wednesdays in your C2GF class and, thanks to you, I've learned about a better way to eat that is good for me.

I've always known that the secret to weight loss was move more and eat less. However, although I knew I should avoid foods that are desserts, I had no idea what "carbs" really were and how much of them could hide in the foods and beverages I consume until you showed us the way. I've always thought there should be an easier, healthy, no magic pills or potions way to weight loss and you've taught me that.

You always tell us you are not an M.D., not a Ph.D., not an N.D., nor an R.D. You say you are a "No D" - Laura there is no "D" in "Success."

Thank YOU for teaching, sharing, and living what you know; you've helped more people than you will ever know!

Gloria

Hola, Laura!

I remember the very first time that I met you at the Y and the first thought that came to my head was, this lady is doing promotion for her own convenience, she comes from a different life style and different social level, why does she want to help others? But through the weeks I was in your C2GF class, I changed my mind—how wrong I was …

I saw in your eyes that you are a genuine person, you had your eyes watering when you told us that we were wonderful people, this is why I have to be honest.

I learned a lot in your group class, but the most important thing that I like was that we can talk without any prejudice about diet, weight, food, exercise, and who loses or gains weight without being criticized, because we all are in the same boat.

In the past, sometimes my self-esteem was a little low due to my weight or my appearance, but since I'm reading your book and your articles on motivation, I have changed.

I said IF LAURA CAN … I CAN, TOO, I'm going to try to be more strict in what I eat and working out.

Thank you for everything you did for us all.

Magda

Laura:

Just wanted to thank you for all your help and for the quote about change that led off your latest motivational blog post. I am down 126 lbs. after a year of hard work, and have changed in many ways.

Having been morbidly obese, I still have probably another year of effort ahead of me, which I fully embrace, but unfortunately, my friends are having a harder time of it accepting the new me …

Refreshed with a new spirit where my life is more about me, my health, and the new experiences that I am having, my friends are less than excited to share in my journey.

Sure, they are happy about my weight loss, but I can only guess that they have an unspoken disappointment because my existence no longer revolves around eating and drinking with them and living their lives vicariously since I hardly had one of my own. This is a hard and unspoken truth, but one I am having to work through nearly every day in my relationships.

I never thought that my biggest supporters would also become my biggest detractors, but I suppose that change is hard on everyone—especially if they choose to not embrace it. All this said, I will never give up the good fight … I've come too far now to give up, and my new life is exactly that, mine, and mine to live to the fullest.

Thankfully, I am no longer tempted by my old demons.

It's amazing what a sincere lifestyle change, endurance, and patience can do for a person. If we could only bottle this and share it, the world would be a much better place.

Thanks again for sharing the quote, helping motivate me to do this … it was a wise word for me today.

Regards,

R

Dear Laura:

What do I like best about you? YOU! You're genuine, and you deeply care for people. What is great about you is that it is not just for your family and friends—the people you know. You care for people you don't even know! I liked that you don't say everyone HAS TO follow the low-carb way. You let them pick which diet they want but if that isn't working, you find out what they are doing and help them to make it work, however that may be.

What I liked about CTGF is that it gave me the kick in the butt I needed to get going. You gave me the knowledge to make it work.

C2GF was fun. I met a lot of great people and we all got along so well. I looked forward to Wednesday evenings to see everyone and talk, laugh, and, most of all, learn.

Meg

Hi Laura,

I want to thank you for giving me the insight to learn more about eating properly. Since I started listening to you at ECC I find that I am feeling much better all around and have more energy. I have lost weight and I do notice that if I "cheat" I gain weight by a few ounces or pounds. I do have to walk more. It is not from lack of desire but more because I am trying to balance full time work, family, kids, and my own business.

I was unable to attend most of the classes either b/c of business or family commitments, but I really got my money's worth for the few classes that I did attend.

Kudos to you for sharing your story and encouraging others to do it, too. Keep on trucking; you help make a tremendous difference in people's lives.

Kay

Dear Laura:

I'm a seventy-five-year old Italian immigrant male who found the motivation through working with you to lose forty pounds so I could keep up with my younger buddies moose hunting in Montana.

Thank you so much for helping me achieve my weight loss, wellness, and moose hunting goals!

Tom

Dear Laura:

Absolutely love the way you motivate, write, and reach out to your participants long after your C2GF classes are over.

I can hear you talking to me as if you were standing right before me or as if we ran into one another on the street …

Keep your motivational articles comin'!

Cyn

Hi Laura,

I just wanted to thank you for all you are doing for all of us.

I know I am the "twig" of the group. It is strange to even be called that—it's a first.

But for me, your C2GF class has been so great. I have been accomplishing every one of my personal goals for the past two months because of your motivational help. That is something I rarely do.

I am now much more fit and healthier than I was when I started your class and I am grateful for that. Your program works for sure, even if my numbers don't show it!

I am so grateful for what you are doing!

Sincerely,

Bet

Laura,

As I count the many blessings received during the past year, meeting you is one of those good fortunes.

Your passion for helping others become healthy is an example to be followed. Thank you for what you have taught me this year. May the New Year be your best year yet. May it bring you only good things. May it be the year you are allowed to shine the brightest yet!

Thank you for all you do.

Love,

Lisa

Dear Laura,

June 2 is the day I changed my life FOREVER!

In my last job, I was an overweight employee on the NASA Space Shuttle program where I helped design the largest rocket in the world—the big orange external fuel tank on Space Shuttle missions—but I'm no rocket scientist when it comes to successfully launching a healthy eating and exercise program for myself. My missions always failed. YOU, Laura, are the genius!

I came across your radio show, "The Laura Dion-Jones Show" on a Wed. afternoon in May or April on WRMN 1410 AM. You were telling how you'd lost 150-pounds in two and a half years. I thought that was great— but then you said, "And I've kept it off for nine years!" WOW! I've never known anyone that lost a lot of weight and was able to KEEP it off. So you got my attention.

I just HAD to know how you did it and are doing it. I was so sick of the low-fat, low-calorie, low-taste, unsatisfying diets I'd been on in the past, which I couldn't maintain.

I contacted you via e-mail that day and you told me about your Commit To Get Fit program. I signed up immediately for the next session that started that June 2nd.

From that day forward I haven't looked back. In your C2GF, you taught me that, like your own metabolic system, I just cannot metabolize high carbohydrates in my diet.

I listened to your life story and thought, *She's talking about me! Why not give it a try? What do I have to lose, except lots of weight?* You, Laura, are a walking success story. I thought, *I can be too!* I then read your book, *Commit to Get Fit* several times and got the Atkins new book and dove in.

I added working out from ten to fifteen minutes a day to sixty minutes and some days ninety. I've lived for your "thinspirational" motivational talks after weigh-in every Wednesday. I did what you suggested and have lost thirty pounds. I feel so much better.

You have no idea how much you've helped me (and a lot of others) change my life for the better. It's a GOD thing that I met you.

You're the genius rocket scientist, here, Laura! You have it figured out. You've had **mission success!** And now so do I.

Sincerely,

J.

Notes

Notes

Notes

Notes

www.ingramcontent.com/pod-product-compliance
Lightning Source LLC
Chambersburg PA
CBHW070800280326
41934CB00012B/2988